D0428792

THROUGH THE FIRE & THROUGH THE WATER

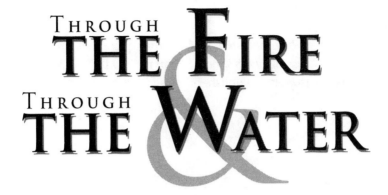

THROUGH THE FIRE & THROUGH THE WATER

My Triumph Over Cancer

Dr. Betty R. Price

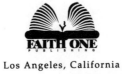

Los Angeles, California

Unless otherwise indicated, all Scripture quotations are taken from *The New King James Version.* Copyright © 1979, 1980, 1982, Thomas Nelson, Inc., Publishers. Used by Permission.

Through The Fire And Through The Water
My Triumph Over Cancer
ISBN 1-883798-20-5
Copyright © 1997 by
Betty R. Price, D.D.
P.O. Box 90000
Los Angeles, CA 90009

Published by Faith One Publishing
7901 South Vermont Avenue
Los Angeles, CA 90044

*"...We went through fire
and through water;*

*But You brought us out
to rich fulfillment."*

- Psalm 66:12 (NKJV)

I dedicate this book to my husband, Fred,
and to my children,
Angela, Cheryl, Stephanie, and Frederick,
who went through the fire and through the
water with me.

—*Betty R. Price*

Acknowledgments

First, I want to give all the praise and honor to God for sending His Word which heals. I thank Him for having provided me with such wonderful doctors and nurses, whose compassion, skill, knowledge, and expertise were available to assist me in my fight against cancer. Words cannot express my appreciation to them for their genuine concern and care.

I thank God for the love expressed to me by my sister Stella, and my brothers Sylvester, Wallace, Baltimore, and Leonard throughout this attack on my health. I particularly want to thank my sons-in-law Michael Evans, Allen Crabbe, and Danon Buchanan for their love and support, as well as my mother-in-law, Mrs. Winifred Price. Words are inadequate to express my great appreciation for the support and prayers of my many relatives and friends. They are all truly special to me, and I thank God for them.

I praise God for having blessed me and my husband with the wonderful congregation of Crenshaw Christian Center and for the Ever Increasing Faith TV viewers — our extended family. I am also grateful to God for having given my husband and me such wonderful brothers and sisters in Christ in the ministry. Their words of encouragement and prayerful support helped to undergird our faith.

And finally, I want to thank Pat Hays and Julianne Nachtrab for their editorial assistance in the preparation of this book.

—Betty R. Price

CONTENTS

Foreword

SHOCK, ANGER, and JOY perhaps best describe the range of emotions I felt as a participant in the medical care of Dr. Betty Price during the attack of cancer upon her body. Dr. Betty, as she is often called by members of the church that her husband pastors, is a gracious, beautiful lady whose family I have come to know, love, and respect during my many years as a member of Crenshaw Christian Center, but particularly during the time this crisis invaded the Price family.

Shock was what I felt when the diagnosis was finally made. I never dreamt that the offender would be a lymphoma — a malignant tumor that, ironically, courses out of the very tissue that is designed to protect the human body from infection and disease.

Then came **anger** because, once the diagnosis was clear, I was the one who had to be the bearer of this dreaded news to an unsuspecting family — my very own pastor and the first lady of my church.

Finally, there was **joy**, knowing they knew the real Healer and how to stand on the Word of God in faith for healing because God is faithful and an ever-present help in a time of need.

Early in the course of Dr. Betty's treatment, I had become acquainted with a nutritional program fostered by a gentleman known as the "Juiceman," and the concept of live foods, including the juicing of fresh fruits and vegetables as a way of achieving and maintaining a healthy body. I presented this data to the Prices. I now believe, along with Dr. Betty, that had she been miraculously or instantly healed, she would not be practicing today the good health habits she has since developed (including proper nutrition, good bowel care, use of food supplements, and exclusion of excess coffee).

During the course of her treatment, I presented a letter to Dr. Betty on the "personality" of the cancer (see Appendix IV) violating her body. I described its nature, characteristics, and suggested she spiritually take authority over these characteristics and this satanic attack trying to engulf her. I had no doubt she knew how to do this, nor any doubt that she would.

Finally acknowledging that chemotherapy and irradiation were the way for her to go, Dr. Betty accepted the course laid out for her. Being informed of what she was going to have to face — loss of hair, discomfort, and anguish — she put her hands to the plow without a whine or a complaint. I visited Dr. Betty every week during the entire time of her illness. Each time I saw her, she greeted me with a smile and a firm handshake. Her faith and ability to endure pain were amazing, and I was often reminded of what Jesus endured on the cross for the joy of bringing many sons and daughters to the heavenly Father. She knew she was being watched and that faith — her faith — was on trial.

Having practiced medicine as an internist for the past 18 years, I have seen very few people who were able to walk through the fire and through the water as bravely as Betty Price. She followed James 1:2-4 to the letter: **My brethren, count it all joy when you fall into various trials, knowing that the testing of your faith produces patience. But let patience have its perfect work, that you may be perfect and complete, lacking nothing.**

While the support of her team — her family, a plethora of relatives and friends, as well as gifted medical practitioners — helped keep her spirit high and kept her fighting when times were bad, she never lost sight of the fact that it was her own determination to do God's Word and her own confidence in the Lord that was going to bring her through.

As you read this great testimony of faith and of what the Lord wrought through modern medicine, just know He is no respecter of persons. I am confident that what the Father God did for Betty Price, He will do for you, if you are willing to take a stand on the uncompromising Word. And I am also confident that Dr. Betty will be the first to tell you so.

If you have a medical situation that needs attention, see your doctor. Do not operate in foolishness or presumption. Use your faith to get over and through the situation. This is what Dr. Betty did. Remember what 1 Corinthians 10:13 says: **No temptation has overtaken you except such as is common to man; but God is faithful, who will not allow you to be** tempted beyond what you are able, but with the temptation will also make the way of escape, that you may be able to bear it.

—William F. Taylor, M.D.

Publisher's Note: Dr. Taylor is a specialist in the field of Internal Medicine. A Born-again, Spirit-filled Believer, Dr. Taylor is a graduate of the Crenshaw Christian Center Ministry Training Institute, with a call to the fivefold ministry offices of Evangelist and Teacher.

1

THROUGH THE FIRE

"Higher" squealed Nicole, my one-year-old granddaughter, as she straddled my leg to get a "horsy ride." Nikki had hopped on top of my right leg that I had crossed over my left knee and I was holding onto her arms while raising her up and down as if she were on a seesaw. Nikki loved it when I gave her these "horsy rides," especially when I would lift her up high. But this particular day I could not lift her very high. My leg began to throb painfully with my every effort to lift her. For days after my right leg ached.

The ministry had a television crusade coming up in Houston, Texas that was scheduled for the last week of May of 1990, which was only a few days away. Since I always spoke at a women's luncheon held during our crusades, I had to go even though I was feeling unusually tired and my leg was continuing to bother me. It was as I was getting dressed for the luncheon that I noticed how swollen my right leg had become. While ministering at the luncheon, I remember telling the women I was there by faith because I did not feel up to par. I was sharing with

1

them the different ways Satan tries to attack and distract you, and how it is important to keep right on doing what God has called you to do regardless of how the devil tries to make you feel or think.

After the luncheon, I returned to our hotel room. Fred, my husband, took a look at my leg and agreed that it was very swollen. I called Dr. Rosetta Bush, a pediatrician from our church, who had come to Texas with us to attend the meetings. She came to our hotel room to examine my leg. She said I should see an internist as soon as I got home. This was on Friday of the Memorial Day weekend.

The next day we flew home. I had never seen an internist before; however, God had placed Dr. William Taylor, a Spirit-filled internist, in our congregation. Since he lived near our daughter Angela, we decided to go directly to Angela's home and then call Dr. Taylor to see if he could come over to take a look at my leg. Dr. Taylor agreed to meet us at Angie's house. After closely examining my leg, Dr. Taylor said it did not look normal. He drew some of my blood to send to the lab. Because it was a holiday weekend, my test results would not be back until late that night; so Fred and I took the opportunity to go home and relax.

When the results did come back, Dr. Taylor called to say my blood tests did not detect any abnormalities. Yet he was not happy leaving me without an answer as to what could be troubling my leg. It was far too swollen for this to have simply been a pulled or strained muscle. The swelling was very odd because, up until just before the crusade, I had been "perfectly healthy" — or so I thought. Fred and I had returned from vacation only a few weeks earlier. We had walked all over London and Paris, and had even traveled to Africa. I felt perfectly fine throughout our entire vacation. In fact, upon our return, I even started an exercise program. So when I had trouble lifting Nikki and began to feel a little pain in my leg, I thought I had just sprained or strained a muscle from all the recent walking and exercising. Even though the pain began to intensify, I prayed and stood on the Word that I was healed as I went about doing my usual tasks as a wife, mother, and help meet to my husband in the ministry.

Dr. Taylor called his friend Dr. Fombé Ndiforchu, a general surgeon, who happened to live next door to us. Dr. Ndiforchu came over to our house to examine my leg. Dr. Ndiforchu insisted I be taken to the hospital immediately. Of course we were not expecting this, but the unusual swelling did look serious. Fred and I had already agreed I was healed; we still felt nothing life-threatening was wrong and that I would be home from the hospital by the next day. During my first night in the hospital, while lying in bed and praying in tongues, I heard in my spirit, **"This sickness is not unto death, but for the glory of God, that the Son of God may be glorified through it"** (John 11:4). At that time I had no idea as to the gravity of my condition, so I did not recognize the sweet, blessed assurance this scripture was to become. I was in the hospital more than a week, undergoing test after test, before the doctors finally were able to determine what the problem was with my leg. Through all of those extremely uncomfortable tests and all of the waiting, I was never anxious. I never worried, nor was I fearful. I was at peace the whole time. In fact, my children and I would joke about all the tests.

We could tell the news was not good by the way Dr. Taylor looked when he came into my hospital room. I felt so badly for him because I could tell he did not want to have to give me such news. He had called in several different doctors to consult on my case and had the medical laboratory working around the clock before he had what he believed was the proper diagnosis. "Fred, Angela, and Mrs. Price," he began, "I'm afraid I have some bad news. The MRI shows there is a growth located in your pelvic area; we need to do a biopsy before we can determine whether or not it is malignant. Unfortunately, because of the tumor's location, it will require major surgery just to perform the biopsy. We will have to go through your abdomen to get a good look at the tumor, then take a sample of the tissue, and see what can be done about it."

This certainly was not what we had expected to hear. We both knew that God was in control of our lives and our trust was in Him. We believed this tumor would not be cancerous, but something the doctors could take care of and it would not be long before I would be back on my feet again. I was scheduled for major surgery the very next morning.

I can hardly remember the people coming and going after my surgery because it all remains just a haze of pain. When I awoke from the surgery, I wondered how I would ever live through the pain; my entire body hurt. I took comfort in knowing God was with me, but having that surgery was no fun! I do remember hearing Fred and my children sobbing when they saw me lying in that hospital bed. It was hard for them to see me like that; not even with all of my five childbirths had I ever been so immobilized. It is only natural to cry when you see someone you love hurting. This does not mean you do not have faith; it is just that it hurts to see the person you love in pain. I wanted so much to reach out and comfort my family, but I could not even speak — let alone move.

Fred later told me that he could not help but cry because he hated seeing me like that. He said that for once in my life I was totally helpless. And I really was helpless when I came out of that surgery. I said, "Lord, it is just You and me. You are going to have to take me through this." Despite all the faith Fred had in my complete recovery, he knew his faith could not override my own will and desire.

Again, the news the doctors had to report was not what we expected. "You have an inoperable malignant tumor in your pelvic region," the surgeon informed us when he came to see me the day following my surgery. "It is inoperable because it is attached to a vital nerve ending, muscle, and blood vessels. Chemotherapy, followed by radiation, is what we recommend to treat you for this." Of course my children were in shock; Fred was shocked and confused by such a diagnosis. None of them could understand how this could be happening to me. Again, I wanted so much to reach out and tell them it was okay. I wanted them to know it was only my body that was hurting and I was okay because God is still the same regardless of my condition. Nothing is too hard for God. When you hear the word *cancer*, fear can come over you. I believe fear is what kills many people in this situation — not the cancer! So I wanted to assure them I was not afraid. Physically, I was too weak to respond, but my spirit was strong with trust in the Lord.

Despite my condition, Fred had to leave later that day for San Diego to attend our Men's Fellowship Advance. Plans had already been made, and he knew he had to put into operation what he had been teaching the people for so many years — that God is a very present help in time of need and, if we have faith, He will bring us out on top of every circumstance. My husband had to go through all of this with me and still minister to the congregation, as well as take care of his responsibilities at home and at the church. With God's help he did it — through the entire time it took for me to receive the physical manifestation of my complete recovery and restoration. Fred went to minister to our men just like nothing was trying to threaten my health. He traveled to the Men's Advance, went out to dinner with the Men's Executive Board, and acted on what he believed. When he got back to his hotel room that evening, he prayed in the spirit for about three hours. He said he prayed with tears streaming down his face until he finally got a release in his spirit to cease praying.

While Fred was interceding for me, I was alone in my hospital room. I was feeling very weak and in so much pain that I could not get up, move, or do anything. Suddenly I felt a presence so strong that I knew the Lord had come into my room. I felt strength coming into my body. It was the middle of the night, and here I was reaching up and moving around as the strength of God flowed through me. As suddenly as the presence had come, it was gone — and so was the weakness and most of the pain. I felt stronger than I had since the surgery. I remembered the words I had heard in my spirit that very first night I spent in the hospital. Those words, **"This sickness is not unto death, but for the glory of God, that the Son of God may be glorified through it"** (John 11:4), instantly became very precious to me. They sustained me throughout this attack on my health. I knew in my heart what the devil had meant for my harm, the Lord would turn around to bring glory to His Son, Jesus Christ, our Divine Healer. Just like in the days of old, He had sent His Word and healed me (Psalm 107:20).

I knew from the Word of God that our Father's desire was for me to be healthy. It is silly to think you can somehow be a better witness for Jesus Christ when you are sick than when you are walking in divine health. Sickness and disease does not glorify God. But when you see God's Word as your source and let His Word take precedence over your circumstances, then your faith can tap into the power of God to affect a healing and a cure on your behalf. God will never violate your free will, so your faith permits Him to move on your behalf to bring about the physical manifestation of His declared Word. And it is His Word coming to pass that brings God glory (Romans 4:20). Your healing or cure brings glory to God; this is how we truly glorify our heavenly Father.

If I had died, how would that possibly have glorified our Lord? I believe what the Holy Spirit said to me my first night in the hospital meant Jesus Christ was going to be glorified *through* this attack on my body because I was going to live — *not* that He was glorified *by* it. God does not put sickness or disease on anyone because there is no sickness or disease in Him. If you study John 11:4 in the original Greek, you will see the word *but*, in this case, implies "that which is contrawise or contrary," and the word *for* translates "for the sake of" or "on behalf of." So, contrary to this sickness bringing death, God was going to see to it that I lived for the sake of bringing glory to His name.

The next day Fred called from San Diego. My voice was much stronger and I could hear how happy he was that I was sounding so much better. We discovered the moment I began to feel my strength returning was just about the same time he was praying for me in the spirit. When Fred returned from the Men's Advance that Saturday evening, I could see the relief on his face when he saw me sitting up in bed. "I don't understand how such a devastating thing could happen to you," he said. He knew I had always tried to live to the very best I knew how for the Lord; so neither of us had an inkling at that time as to how a malignant tumor had developed in my body. But the one thing I did know was nothing was too hard or too big for God, and I believed He would bring me out of this situation. His Word says in Deuteronomy 30:19:

> **"I call heaven and earth as witnesses today against you, that I have set before you life and death, blessing and cursing; therefore choose life, that both you and your descendants may live."**

I chose life; I did not believe the Lord would tell me to choose life and then let me die. I was released to go home a few days later.

Fred and I talked. I told him I did not want to take the chemotherapy or radiation treatments; I was going to believe God for my healing. I told Fred that I did not believe God wanted me to take chemotherapy because it kills your good cells and destroys your body. I said I did not believe God wanted me to put that poison into my body — that was my thinking, *God did not tell me this.* The truth was I had actually gotten into the natural; I was considering the circumstances. I did not want to take these treatments because I had heard and seen the bad things that had happened to people taking chemotherapy and radiation. *God never told me* **not** *to take these treatments.* Instead of carefully considering this option, I just believed I would not have to take the chemotherapy or radiation — that was my decision, based on my own free will. I still do not know why I did not think to trust God to get me through the chemotherapy and radiation without all the ill side effects I knew others suffered. Praise God for His mercy!

See how we can miss God no matter how much we know? I learned later that no matter what you are faced with, you just have to face it. In the 91st Psalm, the Word of God lets you know God does not consider how many other people have died from what you are facing or whatever else happened to someone in your situation — that does not have anything to do with you. The Bible says in Psalm 91:7:

> **A thousand may fall at your side,**
> **And ten thousand at your right hand;**
> **But it shall not come near you.**

Sometimes people allow what they see happen to others wrongly discourage them from maintaining their stand of faith. But you cannot afford to let what may or may not happen to other people discourage you from maintaining your own stand. I am here to tell you that even if I had died, healing is still true because God says so in His Word, and the Word of God is not based on someone's experience — or lack of it.

Looking back, I now realize I had allowed what I saw others go through to influence my thinking regarding treatments. My own sweet, beautiful sister Tina had died of stomach cancer when she was only 34 years of age. She had undergone a series of treatments which failed to halt the spread of this disease. I vividly remember the burn marks on her body.

July, August, and September came and went. Even though I had not returned to working at the church, I still attended our services on Sundays. My leg was not as swollen as it had been before the surgery, but it was still quite sensitive and painful, and I had some difficulty walking. In September, our youngest daughter, Stephanie, got married to a young man who had grown up with her in our church. I was grateful I was able to take part in their wedding. But even more so, I was grateful to the Lord that all of my girls had married good Christian men, who loved God and would take care of them. Now all of our three girls and their husbands were working with us in the ministry.

October came and went. The growth was getting larger, and the pain more intense as it grew. As the pain grew, so did the letters, books, tapes, and information come to the church with advice for me. I was sent so much information — literally drawers and closets full. Every package was from well-meaning, wonderful people, but there was so much sent that it would have taken me two or three years just to read or listen to all of it. If I had not been standing in faith, I would have died before having the chance to get through all the materials sent! This is why you need to trust in the Lord when you are under attack. For those of you wishing to minister to people, you have such a wonderful desire, but be sure you are led of the Lord before offering, sending, or giving any advice and information to anyone making a stand of faith. Otherwise, you might open the door for Satan to come in with confusion and distractions which could cost someone his or her very life! God's voice is the only voice you want to receive direction from when giving or receiving advice and information.

Thank God for His coming to me again during this time. He spoke these words to my spirit, **Be still, and know that I am God**. I knew this was in the Bible, but I did not know where. When I opened my Bible, I turned to it without even looking it up! I found it in Psalm 46:10. This psalm begins, **God is our refuge and strength, A very present help in trouble**. Over in verse 10 it reads, **Be still, and know that I am God**. That was exactly what I decided to do. I simply could not listen to all the different cures and remedies people were trying to give me. Besides, I already knew what to do and had staked my claim that I believed I was healed by faith according to Mark 11:24. I could not allow anyone's desire to help cause me to waiver in my stand of faith.

If you knew all the people who were trying to help and wanted my attention, you would understand why this point is so very important. One lady flew to Los Angeles with her husband, claiming the Lord had sent her to come and pray for me. I really felt badly for her because she was very upset when she was not able to minister to me during one of our regular Sunday services. Apparently she did not realize that if the Lord really had told her to come and pray for me, then He would have told me as well so I could have been sure we made the appropriate preparations for her. Our church simply is too large for us to stop everything to heed the voice of every person who has something to say on a given Sunday morning. It is not that we do not care, because we love the people God has blessed us to minister to, but it just would not be fair to all the others who have come to worship, hear, and focus on God. It also is not biblical. The Apostle Paul wrote in 1 Corinthians 14:29 to **Let two or three prophets speak, and let the others judge**. He also wrote in verse 40 of that same chapter, **Let all things be done decently and in order**. Our God is a God of Order. Making prior arrangements, or an appointment, would have been **decently and in order**. But this woman, bless her heart, just showed up with her husband to one of our regular Sunday services. Naturally she had a hard time getting to me, so she became really upset. Her husband told her just to forget about it, but she was so worked-up. She kept crying, "I've got to pray for Betty, the Lord told me. My husband told me to forget about it, but Betty is calling for me." Yet I never called for her.

I figured this way, I was going to be still and know the Lord is God. I had already prayed and believed I was healed by faith. I did not need someone else to heal me — God already healed me because I had His Word on it. A lot of people have a need to be the one God uses. This is sad because they are precisely the people God cannot use since they would seek to take all the glory for themselves.

No one person should be so caught up in being *the* one — Jesus is The Only One. As Christians, we should all be working together, letting Him get all the glory! If you are under attack, you cannot afford to take your focus off of God as your source. So there is a very thin line you have to draw between being responsible and seeking the help you need and seeing or allowing anything or anyone to be your source. But you have got to draw it in order to keep things right before God. *Be sure to seek the help you need*, but also ask yourself, "Whom do I see as my source? Who is going to get the glory in my doing this?" Seek God's guidance and direction. Then you will know where to draw that line.

In the middle of October, our Women's Fellowship sponsors our annual women's luncheon, where I minister to the wonderful ladies of our congregation. I particularly wanted this opportunity to speak to our women because of the many rumors that were now circulating concerning my condition. I wanted them to be assured of my stand of faith that I knew would pull me through this attack on my body. After sharing the Word and assuring the ladies I would see them at our next annual luncheon (because I believed I was healed based on Mark 11:24), many of the women openly cried. I could tell some of them did not believe I would make it through to the next year. They were so devastated by the news that they could not believe the faith part of my message — which was the whole point! I was just saying what God says; He calls you healed when you do not yet have the physical manifestation. *He calls those things that be not as though they were; but He does not call those things that be as though they were not.* I did not deny the attack raging in my body, but I did not talk about it either. I talked about and focused on my healing. *This is the way faith talks and the way faith works.* I wanted the ladies to be in agreement and grow with me through this experience, but many could not see past my doctor's report. As Ministers of the Gospel, we have so much work to do — many times right in our own churches!

About this time, I began taking intensely hot baths to soothe my leg and relieve some of the pain, as well as strong pain-killing medication. All the while, I continued my confessions that I believed I was healed according to God's Word. My husband and children were jewels. They encouraged me and confessed the Word with me. I was told that whenever anyone asked about me, they would always say, "She's doing fine." They did not say I *felt* fine, but that I was "doing" fine because *I believed I was healed.* I know it was hard for them to watch me hobbling around and to see me in constant pain.

There were also two absolutely wonderful women who worked for us, Susana and Anna. They did all the cleaning, washing, and cooking for Fred, Frederick and Fred's mother, who lives with us. I was particularly grateful for Susana, who worked late nearly every day and made herself available to my every need. I will never forget her kindness, gentleness, and concern for me during this time.

I also will never forget the love and continual comfort of one particular dear friend, Argie Taylor.

The Lord had brought her back into my life just before this attack, and she spent a good deal of time with me throughout this ordeal. She came to see me almost every day while I was both in the hospital and at home, praying with me and encouraging me. Argie and I had been close during the early years of Fred's first full pastorate at the West Washington Community Church. Shortly after we moved to our Inglewood facility, we lost contact with one another for several years. She had been called into the ministry and was kept very busy, as was I. She was truly a special blessing to me.

November came and left with no change in my condition, except that the tumor continued to grow and become more painful. It was not so funny at the time, but we all laugh now about the rumor that got started when I was on our ministry tour of Greece and the Mediterranean Sea. Our ministry tours are planned way in advance, and many people from across the country had planned to go on this trip with us. We did not want to disappoint them, or cause them too much of an inconvenience by canceling the tour because of my challenge. So I decided to go with the team. I did not feel like going, but Fred and the girls said, "You don't feel well at home, so you might as well not feel well in Greece." My doctors said it was okay, so I went along. We do not know how the rumor got started, but it was said I became seriously ill in Greece and had to be hospitalized. This was entirely false; there was no such hospitalization. I did not have the manifestation of my healing at that time and I did not feel well, but I used wisdom.

While the tourists went on their excursions, I rested. I was not hospitalized at all during the trip; so you cannot always believe what you hear through the grapevine.

In December, Fred and I usually take a week's vacation out of the city just before the holidays, which we like to spend at home with our family. We particularly enjoy Hawaii in December but, because of my condition, we decided to go some place nearby. Even still, I was in such discomfort that we had to cut short our vacation week. I needed the solace of my own bathroom, bedroom, and prayer closet. Little did I know the last Sunday in December of 1990 was to be the last time I would be able to be in church until Resurrection Sunday ("Easter Day") in April of 1991, and that my greatest challenges were still ahead of me.

2

AND THROUGH THE FIRE

By the first part of January, I could actually feel the growth protruding along my right side. I began using a wheelchair to get around the house, and I was taking hot baths more and more often, even though they were becoming less and less effective. This was when Psalm 23:4 truly became real to me:

> Yea, though I walk through the valley of the
> shadow of death,
> I will fear no evil;
> For You are with me;
> Your rod and Your staff, they comfort me.

At times the pain was overwhelming, and I could see no end in sight. It was like I was in a dark tunnel with no light at either end. I felt as though I was in utter darkness. All I knew was the Lord was with me because He gave me His Word on it in Hebrews 13:5:

> ...For He Himself has said, "I will never leave
> you nor forsake you."

So I would say, **"Yea, though I walk through the valley of the shadow of death, I *will* fear no evil."** I knew fear was a matter of choice. I could have willed to fear evil, but I did not. I believed I was healed and I never saw myself as dead. I saw myself as completely healed and restored to perfect health. Yes, I was feeling badly, but I looked to the Word and not at how I felt or what I saw in the mirror. I also took refuge in Psalm 118:17:

> **I shall not die, but live,**
> **And declare the works of the LORD.**

It was so very dark, but Proverbs 3:5-6 told me:

> **Trust in the LORD with all your heart,**
> **And lean not on your own understanding;**
> **In all your ways acknowledge Him,**
> **And He shall direct your paths.**

It did not matter that I did not understand the why, the how, and the wherefore of this attack on my health. My trust was in God, and I believed with all my heart that He would tell me what I needed to know. Thank God I knew better than to be blinded by the darkness. I continued to thank Him for His promises in His Word and the light they shed in that black tunnel.

I received heart-warming and encouraging letters from people all around the world telling me they were praying for my healing — so many letters from my beautiful Christian brothers and sisters who wanted me to know they were standing with me. The love expressed in those letters was really a comfort to me. There are no words I could ever say that would adequately express what those letters and words of encouragement meant to me. They helped to keep my spirits high many a day. But in the middle of the night, I had to take comfort in prayer and the Word of God. I found that the middle of the night is particularly hard when you are going through a serious illness or mental depression because the rest of your household is asleep. You are left all alone with your thoughts and the pain. Thank God for His desire to fellowship with us in prayer and the consolation of His Word.

It was the Hagins who were instrumental in getting me to begin the chemotherapy treatments. Kenneth and Oretha Hagin kept in constant contact with us, offering words of encouragement and prayers. Doug Jones, who taught Healing School at their Rhema Bible School in Tulsa, Oklahoma, heard from a cancer patient who was attending the healing school about a doctor in the Los Angeles area who had achieved good success with a machine that could destroy cancerous tumors without harming the good cells around it. Doug encouraged Fred to consult with this physician, Dr. Kenneth Tokita, to see if something could be done to help me. Fred made an appointment for us to meet with Dr. Tokita. After reviewing the medical reports from my previous doctors, Dr. Tokita said his treatment did not work on the type of tumor that had invaded my body, which was called a lymphoma. His machine was not a "magic cure-all," as he put it. Dr. Tokita told us the very same thing my previous doctors had said, that intensive chemotherapy followed by extensive radiation was the appropriate treatment for this condition. Since by this time the pain really had arrested my attention, I agreed to start chemotherapy right away.

Thank God Dr. Tokita's opinion finally convinced me to take action against the tumor now protruding from my right side. Otherwise, being a "dummy," I might have died. Then God would have been blamed for my death when it was not His doing. God had made a way of escape, but it was up to me to trust Him through it. I heard some people were surprised when they learned I was taking medication and was going to undergo chemotherapy and radiation treatments. They seemed to think having faith means you do not utilize what God has made available to you. We never said you do not take medication when you are operating in faith. If you read Fred's very first book, *How Faith Works*, he specifically mentions that taking medication has nothing to do with your faith; nor does taking medication and consulting with doctors negate your faith. Your faith is to be based on believing you have received what you have asked God for. In the meantime, until you have the physical manifestation of what is already yours in the spirit realm, you are going to experience the symptoms. Medication only helps you deal with the symptoms; you need the medication to help keep you from suffering, so take it! I did!

Before beginning the chemotherapy treatments, Dr. Peter Boasberg, the oncologist I had been referred to, told me about some of the side effects, which I already knew. He said chemotherapy would cause me to lose all of my hair, I would be nauseated a great deal of the time, I would feel tired and weak, and I would lose more weight. But if I got through the first four treatments, then I would be able to take all the treatments. I was determined that, with God's help, I was going to make it through all twelve of those treatments just fine and on schedule.

When I went in to get my check-up before starting the chemotherapy, I could not walk. I needed help getting in and out of the car and I had to use a wheelchair. I could not move my legs, so I was not able to get myself onto the table to take the MRI. Several doctors had to come and put me up on the table to take the MRI, and had to anesthetize me due to the pain — that is how bad I had gotten! The tumor had grown from my pelvis all the way up to my navel and was also growing down my leg. So I could not move my legs.

But after just one week, just one treatment, the chemotherapy had cut the tumor down so I could walk. My doctors were amazed, and I praised God. During the subsequent examination, the oncologist could not even feel the tumor! It had not totally gone, but at least the doctor could not feel it. Now I could get around better — just that quick! God was honoring His Word. When my doctor called to check on me, he said I was doing better than 90 percent of his patients. God was definitely moving through these treatments.

For the next eleven weeks, I went to Dr. Boasberg's office to get my weekly dose of chemotherapy. Just as he had forewarned me, the chemotherapy treatments made me nauseated, weak, and tired. My face became swollen, my skin darkened several shades, and sores broke out in my mouth. It would take me an hour and a half just to get down a little food. But every single one of my blood tests, which the lab would take to make sure my body was handling the treatments sufficiently, came out fine. I never had to postpone any of the treatments. The nurse, who checked my blood every week, would always come back to me saying, "Amazing blood."

Nevertheless, the treatments were very, very hard. I stayed strong by confessing **I can do all things through Christ who strengthens me** (Philippians 4:13). When I would awake in the middle of the night in pain, I would spend that time talking to the Lord. I prayed to the Lord to get me through, and I confessed that my body would not reject the medicine but would allow the medication do what it was supposed to do. I would declare, based upon Psalm 91:10 and 1 Peter 2:24:

> "No evil shall befall me, nor shall any plague come near my dwelling; I am healed by Jesus' stripes so every cell in my body is normal and every organ in my body is functioning properly."

I know it was God's Word that helped me make it through those treatments as well as I did. The nurse, who administered the shots, said it was amazing I did not experience some of the really bad side effects, such as severe anemia or an allergic reaction, due to the heavy doses I was taking. Like I said before, every time she would check my blood, she would come back shaking her head in disbelief and saying, "Amazing blood."

So I want to encourage anyone who might be facing or taking chemotherapy. Get all the treatments you need and stick with those treatments for as long as your doctor advises. Believe God to see you through. I have heard so many tragic stories of people who started on chemotherapy and, because it was so difficult, they did not continue and so they died. I call taking chemotherapy — or whatever you need to do to get well — "possessing the land." God has already healed you, but you have to do certain things. Find out what your part is in your healing and then, if you do your part, God will do His part. Diligently doing those things which you need to do is what I call, "possessing the land." If you take a look at the three Hebrew boys, Shadrach, Meshach, and Abed-Nego, God could have delivered them from the fiery furnace, but He delivered them *through* it (Daniel 3). That was how God let them know He was with them. And often times, that is how He will let you know He is with you.

I never allowed fear to overtake me. My spirit man and my soulish man stayed strong throughout this entire ordeal because of the Word I already had in me. I kept my thoughts and confessions in line with the Word of God. I remembered and confessed Proverbs 4:20-23:

> My son, give attention to my words;
> Incline your ear to my sayings.
> Do not let them depart from your eyes;
> Keep them in the midst of your heart;
> For they are life to those who find them,
> And health to all their flesh.
> Keep your heart with all diligence,
> For out of it spring the issues of life.

No matter what the doctors or anyone else would try to say, I knew God was with me — I had His Word on it in Hebrews 13:5. So I always looked at the *end* of this condition, remembering Psalm 71:20-21:

> You, who have shown me great and severe
>   troubles,
> Shall revive me again,
> And bring me up again from the depths of the
>   earth.
> You shall increase my greatness,
> And comfort me on every side.

Confessing Psalm 138:7-8 also kept me confident in the reality of my healing:

> Though I walk in the midst of trouble, You
>   will revive me;
> You will stretch out Your hand
> Against the wrath of my enemies,
> And Your right hand will save me.
> The LORD will perfect that which concerns me;

**Your mercy, O LORD, endures forever;
Do not forsake the works of Your hands.**

I never looked at how I felt and what I was
going through. *I only looked at the end.* That is what
you have to do. Otherwise, your circumstances can
be overwhelming. You have to forever be **casting
down arguments and every high thing that exalts
itself against the knowledge of God, bringing
every thought into captivity to the obedience of
Christ** (2 Corinthians 10:5). You have to do this
because Satan has access to your mind and he feeds
a million thoughts a minute to your mind. He will
make sure you see and hear about all the bad that
has happened to everyone else.

I am no different than you. Every step I made,
Satan told me negative things were going to happen.
He made sure I knew all about the six or seven people
who had died since I first learned of this attack on my
body. I remember how he tried to taunt me when I
was posing for our annual Christmas portrait we
send out to all of our congregation and television
audience. I had just gotten the news about the cancer
attacking my body and this year, of all years, it
was decided I would pose with flowers all around
me. All the while I was posing for that picture, the
devil was telling me that they were going to use
that shot of me on my funeral program. But I
fought back with the Word of God. The Bible lets
us know in 2 Corinthians 5:8 that to be absent from
the body is to be present with the Lord, and this is
what I used to help me back down the fear Satan was

27

trying to instill in me. You have to be bold enough to talk back to the devil. That is what I did. I said, "Devil, it does not matter, because to be absent from the body is to be present with the Lord. But I believe God, so I am not going to die."

One evening, after about the fourth session of chemotherapy, I was sitting in a chair combing my hair. When I looked at my comb and saw that half of my hair had come out, I knew it would not be long before I would be as bald as could be. My daughter Angela happened to call at that time, and she began feeling sorry for me. I said to her, "Angela, don't feel bad because I don't feel bad. It will give me a rest from rolling my hair and sleeping on rollers." I did not allow my hair loss to get me upset or discouraged because I knew it was only temporary, like all the other symptoms and pain I was experiencing. I had the assurance of 2 Corinthians 4:18: **while we do not look at the things which are seen, but at the things which are not seen. For the things which are seen are temporary, but the things which are not seen are eternal.** I just called my hairdresser and told her I would not be coming for an appointment because I did not have any hair to style. Since turbans had always been my favorite hair cover-up when I had curlers in my hair that I did not want to be seen, I decided they would be my choice for covering my bald head. Fred does not like wigs, so I chose turbans instead. I had them in all colors and styles to match different outfits. At least I did not have to be concerned about rolling my hair at night because

I did not have any hair to roll! There is always a blessing in everything, if you just look for it.

After the chemotherapy, I had to go through radiation five times a week for five weeks. Now, whenever I hear of anyone having to go through chemotherapy or radiation, my heart really goes out to them because I know what it is like to go through these treatments. If you are going through treatments like this, I encourage you to keep your faith in God because He is an ever-present help in time of need and He is always faithful to keep His Word. Know that you can do all things through Christ who strengthens you (Philippians 4:13). I am truly thankful that God led me to undergo these treatments despite how hard it was — and it was hard, but these treatments helped save my life. I stood on the Word given to the prophet Jeremiah.

Jeremiah 30:17:

> **For I will restore health to you**
> **And heal you of your wounds, says the LORD,...**

I continued traveling with my husband during the chemotherapy and radiation treatments. No matter how weak I looked and how badly I felt, Fred and the girls always wanted me with them. We would have to get a wheelchair at the airport, but I still would go. Often I would share my testimony, along with ministry of the Word, at the luncheons and meetings held during our ministry crusades, as well as pray for the sick. Even when I had to sit down to share the Word, I went on because God's Word was still the same regardless of how I was feeling or the way I looked. The devil tried to bombard my mind and say, "Well, you might not even make it and you are up here preaching to these people and telling them what God will do." I had to remind the devil that God's Word is the same whether I made it or not. God honored His Word and gave me the strength to do all I had to do to get through. At the close of the meetings, different people would come and tell me they were going through a similar situation and my testimony had inspired and encouraged them. By the time the chemotherapy was finished, I was walking pretty good and the pain was not nearly as severe. In fact, the pain was being managed quite well through medication. I started going to church again, and a lot of our members were surprised when Fred called out from the pulpit, "Lazarus, come forth," and I walked up to the pulpit on Resurrection ("Easter") Sunday in 1991.

Just about the time I had completed the radiation treatments, my hair had started growing back, but my face was still a little swollen. It took several months before the swelling disappeared completely and my skin returned to its normal color. The sores in my mouth, caused by the chemotherapy treatments, also disappeared and food once again had a taste to it. This increased my appetite some, but my desire for food did not fully return until about two years after my chemotherapy and radiation treatments because the strong medication I was taking kept my stomach feeling topsy-turvy. Then the pain in my hip area returned — and returned with a vengeance!

3

THROUGH THE WATER

Although I was still feeling the devastating effects of the assault on my body from the tumor, the surgery, the chemotherapy, and finally the radiation treatments, I was thrilled when Dr. Taylor told me the latest MRI, taken in October of 1991, showed no traces of cancer in my body. I was scheduled to take another MRI a few weeks later. The doctors primarily wanted to review the extent of the damage done to my thigh bone by the tumor and the radiation treatments, particularly since I was still experiencing quite a lot of pain in the hip area where the tumor had been. The MRI revealed that the tumor had been destroyed, but my femur bone had flattened in the process. "But it should straighten itself out and the pain should go away in about four months," said one of the doctors reviewing my case. I was given strong medication to control the pain and physical therapy was recommended to speed up the restoration of my femur bone.

One day, as I was waiting in front of the hospital while Angela went to get her car from the parking garage, I was pleasantly surprised by two young men who called out to me "Lady, we sure do like your haircut!" as they drove by. My hair was just beginning to grow back, but it was still very short and close to my skull. I wore it slicked down around my face and the back of my neck. Although I thanked them, I received their compliment as being words of encouragement from the Lord. It is wonderful how the Lord will take any opportunity to encourage us when we need it the most. So when our son Frederick later asked me to take him to the local drugstore to get some supplies he needed for a school project, I did not put on my turban. As we were leaving our home Frederick said, "Mom, you forgot your turban." I said, "No, Frederick, I did not forget about it. I am just tired of turbans." Because of the encouraging words the Lord spoke through those young men, I decided I would wear that hairstyle in public.

Four months passed and the pain in my hip was still there, as was the limp — even with the extensive, painful physical therapy. The MRI taken in January of 1992 revealed that the radiation had actually eaten away the entire hip socket so I had bone rubbing against bone. This explained why I was in so much pain. Dr. Taylor made an appointment for me to see Dr. Douglas Garland, an orthopedic surgeon, who told me right from the start that I needed to have hip replacement surgery in order to correct the situation. "After surgery," Dr. Garland stated, "you should not have any more pain, and your walking will be much better."

After what I had gone through with the previous surgery, my mind totally rejected another major operation. I said, "No, I am not having any more surgeries. I am going to believe God." Once again, this was me talking. *I* said, "No way, God, I am going to believe Your Word." I continued on with the physical therapy — smiling, limping, hurting, and believing God for my complete healing. I could not believe I was facing another major battle right on the heels of one of the worst times in my life.

During one of the particularly painful physical therapy sessions, I began to cry. This was the only time I felt a little sorry for myself. The therapist, who had always encouraged me and told me how brave she thought I had been throughout this ordeal, also began to cry. "I know God is with me, and He will bring me out of this some way," I said to Ann, as she massaged my leg. "It is just that right now I feel like crying because I am tired of hurting." There we were, both crying. But crying does not help anything. I do not ever want anyone to feel sorry and cry for me again because that simply is not going to help. Once I had a good cry, I became more resolved than ever to believe God. He had proven Himself faithful to His Word.

James 1:2-4 then came to my remembrance:

> My brethren, count it all joy when you fall into various trials,
> knowing that the testing of your faith produces patience.
> But let patience have its perfect work, that you may be perfect and complete, lacking nothing.

The Bible says we are to **count it all joy** — it does not say *it is* joy! *Count* means "to act like it is," and the word *patience* means "endurance." This Scripture says your endurance is built up while you are going through these various trials. So I had to do what God says; I had to count it all joy. I could not afford to feel sorry for myself and continue to cry. Notice that James wrote, "*When* you fall into various trials." He did not write, "*If* you fall into various trials." What I was experiencing was simply a trial I had to endure. We all will fall into, or be faced with, various trials. It is not the various trials that really matter, but what you do with them and in the midst of them. The Word of God assures us in 1 Corinthians 10:13:

> No temptation has overtaken you except such as is common to man; but God is faithful, who will not allow you to be tempted beyond what you are able, but with the temptation will also make the way of escape, that you may be able to bear it.

God's Word is alive and it works — I could see where God had made a way of escape in my life countless times before. I became sold out to what the Bible declares in 1 John 5:4:

> For whatever is born of God overcomes the world. And this is the victory that has overcome the world — our faith.

I heard many people were questioning why it was taking so long for me to receive the manifestation of my complete healing, and why I had to endure surgery, treatments, and medication. Apparently they thought I would be healed overnight just because I am married to Fred Price. They could not believe it was taking so long. "Why are you not healed already?" they would ask. "Why is it taking you so long?" These people really did not understand what they were saying. *I was already healed by faith.* I believed I was healed the minute I prayed according to Mark 11:24: **...whatever things you ask when you pray, believe that you receive them, and you will have them**. This is what many people do not understand about faith. You have to believe you have received what you have prayed for the minute you pray for it — then you shall have it. No one knows how long you will have to wait for the physical manifestation. But it is not up to you to dwell on when it will come to pass in the natural. It is up to you only to believe you have received your healing when you prayed and asked God for it.

Some people also misconstrue "having faith" to mean you will not have to go through any trials. They do not understand that you do have what you have prayed for — you have it by faith — but you are going to have to **Fight the good fight of faith** (1 Timothy 6:12) and "possess the land." The Old Testament gives us a perfect example of this. God had given the children of Israel the land, but it was up to them to possess it. Everyone except Joshua and Caleb failed to enter into the land because they failed to believe God's Word over their circumstances (Numbers 13). If you do not believe your prayer has been answered the second you prayed your prayer of faith, then you will never take the land. Your confession does not mean your desire is going to come overnight, but it *will come* in time.

While we are waiting, we can take comfort in the fact that God is not concerned about His Word coming to pass. John 11:6 says when Jesus heard Lazarus was sick, Jesus stayed two more days in the place where He was. Jesus did not go running to Lazarus' side. Why? Because Jesus had confidence in His Word. He wanted Mary, Martha, and all of His disciples to have this same confidence. Jesus knew Lazarus' healing was already ensured by the power of the Holy Spirit. He wants us to know that our know knows this same thing so that, having done all, we can still stand — even in the face of death!

"The orthopedic doctor told you that you would not have any more pain once you have the hip surgery," were the words I heard in my spirit as the Holy Spirit ministered to me during one of my morning prayer sessions. I was complaining to Him about how long it was taking for the healing of my hip to be manifested. This was just before Fred was to leave for Africa to minister with Archbishop Benson Idahosa in Nigeria. Angela and her husband, Mike, were going with him. I did not even consider making the trip. Plans had been made way in advance and, although Fred had thought of canceling the trip because of my condition, I insisted he go because I knew Archbishop Idahosa was really looking forward to his coming. He even had made arrangements for Fred to meet with a number of other African ministers so they could get some exposure to the "Word of Faith."

I had been on Percodan, a strong pain-killing medication, for about a year. Even though it did not take away the discomfort entirely, it at least made the pain bearable. I remembered the orthopedic surgeon telling me, "You need to get off that stuff," during my first office visit. "I would rather operate on you than see you stay on that," he said. Thinking back on this conversation, I said to myself, "Dr. Garland is right; I should not have to take this medication the rest of my life to keep me going." In addition to the Percodan, I was taking a couple of other medications for the inflammation. Taking all of those pills made my stomach so upset that I could not eat properly, which meant I could not gain the weight I had lost. All of my size ten clothes were now way too big, and I was now into dress size six.

The day before Fred was to leave for Africa on the 6th of February in 1992, I took myself off of the Percodan. That night I was fine, so I thought I had done the right thing. The next morning I woke up with the worst headache I had ever had in my entire life. I felt like the top of my head was going to come off. I thought some coffee would help me. I was trying to make it into the kitchen to make some coffee when my stomach started heaving. I vomited for hours upon hours. I thought I was going to go into convulsions. I can sympathize with drug addicts; I now have some idea of what it is like going through withdrawal symptoms — and it is absolutely horrible!

When Fred saw the condition I was in, he said, "How can I leave you like this? This is a heck of a time for me to be going to Africa!" He was scheduled to leave that very same morning; in fact, the church van was on the way to pick him up to take him to the airport. He tried to get in touch with Dr. Taylor before he left so he would know what to do, but Dr. Taylor was not available. Fred looked so bewildered; he did not want to go, but he could not stay. There were just too many people involved for him to cancel out at this late of a date. Again, we had to depend upon the Lord to bring us through this trying period.

A short time after Fred left, Dr. Taylor called, and when I told him what I had done, he said, "Oh, no. You cannot do that cold turkey, you have to be detoxed first." He immediately came to our house with the medication I needed. I had to take five different kinds of medication to bring me back to a stable condition. I had to take one of these medications every two hours without fail for the next 24 hours. Even though I was asleep, I had to be awakened and given the medication. Donna Pickens, a dear friend and, at that time, one of our assistant pastors' wives, came and stayed overnight with me because the medicine had to be taken two and three hours apart, both day and night. Angela was on the way to Africa with her father, Cheryl was at home and as big as could be in her last weeks of a complicated pregnancy, and Stephanie needed to be at work. (Since then, Tom and Donna Pickens have established a church in Antelope Valley, California.)

Later, when Fred called from one of his stops, he was able to find out what was wrong and was assured that I would be okay. By the next day, I was feeling much better. The doctor had said it would take me about a week to get back to a stable condition. It only took me a few hours, though, to realize how much the Percodan had helped relieve the pain I had been in for nearly two years. Nothing took the pain away completely, but it helped provide a definite measure of relief. Yet I was determined not to get back on the Percodan. It was then that I decided to follow the advice of the Holy Spirit and the doctor. About four days before Fred returned from his ten-day stay in Africa, I called the doctor and told him of my decision to have hip replacement surgery, saying I still needed to wait until my husband returned home in order for him to be in agreement with me. When Fred got back from Africa, he was in agreement with my decision, and arrangements were made right away for this surgery.

Following the hip replacement surgery, I found the doctor to be absolutely right! The hip replacement took away the excruciating pain and restored my ability to walk with only a slight limp. The hip surgery had not been nearly as bad as the tumor surgery. When Fred came to see me in the hospital, he smiled and said, "You know you almost look like your old self." The doctors had said it would take me about three months to fully recover, but I was up and about in just six weeks. In fact, by April of 1992, I had returned to my full schedule of activity, working at the church, traveling with the ministry,

39

and ministering at various women's retreats and special meetings. Once I got off the Percodan, my stomach returned to normal. Now I actually have to watch myself to make sure I do not gain more weight than I care to. My hair has completely grown back. In fact, I have had it cut several times to keep the style I like.

God is a good, good God. I give Him all the praise and glory! As I have said many times before, the Lord is an ever-present help in time of need, and He is always faithful to keep His Word. I know He was with me through this entire ordeal, and I know He gave me the strength I needed to come out on top and victorious.

4

AND THROUGH THE WATER

Yes, I wanted a miracle. I did not want to go through chemotherapy. I did not want to go through the radiation treatments. I did not want to go through with these treatments because everyone I had seen that had undergone them had a hard time, or they did not make it. They got all burned up and still died. I said to myself, "Well, I do not need to undergo those treatments if they cannot guarantee me that I am going to be healed." So I was slow to take action on my need for chemotherapy and radiation because I wanted to believe for a miracle.

I went for eight months and never received my miracle. As I said before, all the while the tumor kept getting larger and the pain grew worse. It got to the point where I could not walk. I could feel the tumor growing in size up through my abdomen and down the side of my leg. Finally I had to admit, "I guess I am not going to get a miracle." I did not want to be like that story of the man who refused the help God had sent him because he was waiting for a miracle instead. Of course the man died, and when he got to heaven he told God, "Now Lord, I really looked bad because I told all those people You were going to save me." And in essence God said, "Fool, I sent you help and you did not take the way of escape!" So I had to take another look at the chemotherapy and radiation. I did not want to find myself in heaven, asking the Father, "What happened, God? I told everyone You were going to heal me," and then have Him say, "Well, I had chemotherapy and radiation there for you, but you refused to take the way of escape." I finally decided I had better do something and, when I did, I began to see Isaiah 58:8 physically come to pass in my body:

> **Then your light shall break forth like the**
> **morning,**
> **Your healing shall spring forth speedily,**
> **And your righteousness shall go before you;**
> **The glory of the LORD shall be your rear guard.**

Praise God for His mercy and graciousness.

When I read the Gospel accounts of John 5:1-9, when Jesus healed the man at the Pool of Bethesda, and John 9:1-7, of Jesus instructing the blind man to go wash in the Pool of Siloam, I saw both of these men did what Jesus said and they were healed. There are numerous examples of Jesus giving the sick instructions on what to do to be healed. You have to think about that when you are faced with certain situations. Faith is an action. There are some things you may have to do, even though you might not want to, that are not comfortable for you. But you need to be obedient and do as you are advised. I would not be here to write this book if I had not

42

taken the chemotherapy and the radiation treatments. I certainly did not want to undergo those treatments. It was truly a hardship on my body, but I am here to tell you about it. I could not have made it otherwise. Unfortunately, I see too many people failing to get the help they really need. You cannot tell God how to resolve your problems, or how to take care of your situation. You have to believe God *through* your situation.

I think God tries to help people like me, but we do not always listen. Having waited all that time, the tumor caused me to have a problem with my foot that I was able to have taken care of with a little, minor surgery. Had I gone and taken the chemotherapy and radiation treatments when they were first recommended, the tumor would not have gotten so large. The size of the tumor ended up messing up the nerves in my leg. It grew so big it pushed aside the blood vessels and muscles in my hip, causing my leg not to move as it should. As a result of the tumor pressing on the nerve, I developed a hammer toe; one of my toes curved. It pressed against the top of my shoes, especially when I was wearing heels, until I had the worst corn. It was so sore that I just could not put a shoe on that foot anymore.

I went in and had a little surgery to straighten out my toe. They had to break the bone in that toe and put a metal pin through it. The doctor told me that I was going to have terrible pain, like a toothache, and I would not be able to sleep or rest for at least an entire day. He had already given me a prescription for pain medicine that he expected I would need. But not once did I experience any pain from my toe, except when I touched it. Praise God! But had I taken the chemotherapy sooner, I would not have had to go through this minor surgery on my toe, nor would my right leg be injured. Neither should you have to endure damage to your body because you did not respond expediently to an attack on your health.

I can tell you from personal experience that you can make it through chemotherapy and radiation. In fact, I encourage people to undergo these treatments as quickly as possible. Get all the help you need, if you find you have a problem in your body. I would not have had to go through this challenge with my toe, nor have a slight limp with my right leg, had I trusted God to see me through the chemotherapy and radiation treatments before the tumor had the opportunity to grow so big and needlessly harm other areas of my body. Thank God I am alive and He was so merciful. But do not make the same stupid mistakes I made. Get the treatments you need as quickly as possible.

I used Psalm 91 when I was going through chemotherapy and radiation. This Psalm says, **A thousand may fall at your side, And ten thousand at your right hand; But it shall not come near you**. This helped me stand against the fatal side effects of these treatments. This scripture gave me the faith I needed to believe and say, "I don't care what the chemotherapy or radiation has done to someone else, that does not mean it has to do the same to me."

Sometimes when you are going through an attack of cancer, or some other kind of sickness that comes against your body, you may be tempted to think you are not supposed to take medication or get help from a doctor or undergo any treatments or surgery. Just take a moment to really think about this. The devil did not invent doctors, nurses, hospitals, or medication. If you are believing to receive the physical manifestation of your healing by faith, it may be some time before your healing manifests. So you might need to go to a doctor and you might need to take some medication. You may be tempted to say, "Well, I am standing in faith," but are you? Are you really in faith, or are you in denial and fear and in fact acting irresponsibly? I have seen this too many times; it is so unfortunate because many people have lost their lives. It is really tragic. They really were in denial and fear because, if they had been in faith, they would not have died. They were actually thinking, "I do not want to go to the doctor." "I do not want to lose my hair." "I do not want to lose my breast." They think they are just going to make God do something and take care of it for them. But you cannot do that. If there are means available for you to get help, that is what you have to do. You have to use your faith while doing all you know how to do. You have to use your faith to believe God to work through what is available. Isn't it better to be alive, than have a full head of hair and be lying in a coffin?

God has given you a brain and He expects you to use it. Please do not be foolish with your health. Go on and get the help you need because, even if you are standing in faith, you may be doing something to cause your condition. If God just gives you a miracle healing, you might not ever do anything to correct your problem, and it will not be long before you are attacked again.

When the devil tried to tell me that I had done something to somehow deserve this attack on my body, I confessed the first part of Psalm 103:

> **Bless the LORD, O my soul;**
> **And all that is within me, bless His holy name!**
> **Bless the LORD, O my soul,**
> **And forget not all His benefits:**
> **Who forgives all your iniquities,**
> **Who heals all your diseases,**
> **Who redeems your life from destruction,**
> **Who crowns you with lovingkindness and**
>   **tender mercies,**
> **Who satisfies your mouth with good things,**
> **So that your youth is renewed like the eagle's.**

Since the third verse reads, **Who forgives all your iniquities,** I knew that it did not matter what I may or may not have done in the past because He forgives all my iniquities. God is a forgiving God. If you come to Him in true repentance, He will forgive you for *anything* you have done. He forgives you of all your iniquities and heals you of all your diseases. So if you believe the psalmist, how can you die?

Even though God had forgiven me, I still needed to determine if this attack against my health had come as the result of a door that I had somehow left open to Satan. Later I realized, through a book someone had sent me, this was indeed the case. My eating habits had opened the door for Satan to attack my body. I was the type of person who never drank any water. I hated the taste of water, so I did not drink it. I thought, "I'm grown and I do not have to drink water if I do not want to, and I can buy whatever I want to eat." So I did not drink water and I only ate what tasted good to me. What made my situation worse was I really liked coffee. I drank nine cups of coffee a day — three for breakfast, three with lunch, and three with dinner. In this book, I read how coffee pushes the food out of your stomach into your intestines before it is properly digested. This causes elimination problems. Then people go to the drugstore and buy over-the-counter laxatives which are full of toxins.

I also did not eat any fruit, which you need for good nourishment. If I had at least eaten some fruit, I would have gotten some water into my system and some nutrients to sustain a healthy body. Nor did I eat any live food; I never ate any raw food like salads and vegetables. It was not that cooked food was all that bad for me, but more of a case of what I was leaving out of my diet because, when you cook your vegetables, you cook most of the nutrients out of them. So my body did not have the nutrients it needed to maintain healthy cells, fight diseases, and function properly. I believe it was all those toxins building up in my body due to my poor eating habits and elimination troubles that resulted in that tumor forming in my body. It is a marvel I lived 56 good years before I had any real physical challenges in my body. But the body can only take so much. I did not know about good eating habits, but what you do not know can still work against you.

I grew up eating chitterlings, neck bones, red beans, rice, collard greens, pies, bread pudding, and all that good-tasting food. Had God just given me a miracle, I would have never learned the truth about the importance of maintaining a healthy diet. I would have gone right back to eating the same way I had always eaten and, before long, I would have had to be asking for another miracle healing. But thank God this book caught my eye. It had a caption on the cover that talked about increasing your stamina. This really caught my attention because I had always struggled with fatigue. So I started reading this book and learned how I needed to change my diet.

Now I eat fresh fruit in the mornings. I start with a cup of raw apple cider vinegar and warm water, which is really good for you. I mix about two teaspoons of the vinegar with eight ounces of warm water. Then I have a grapefruit or an orange along with an apple. Sometimes I might eat a pear or maybe some melon, when they are in season. A little later on, I will have a banana. This is my breakfast and it fills me up. From what I have read from the book *Fit For Life*, you should eat any kind of fresh fruit you desire up until 12:00 noon. For lunch, I have a green salad with all the green lettuce I can find — except for iceberg lettuce, which does not have any nutritional value. I especially enjoy the romaine lettuce and the butter lettuce, but I like to mix a variety of all the different kinds of green lettuces together. I usually mix a large portion of these greens with some fresh, raw vegetables. I make my own dressing by mixing some olive or canola oil with lemon juice, fresh garlic, and some herb seasonings. I might have either bread or toast along with my big salad, if I do not have a baked white or sweet potato. You could substitute the baked potato with a light, vegetarian soup. If I get hungry before dinner, I will have some more fruit, but I wait until three hours after my lunch and am sure I give myself a good 45 minutes to an hour after finishing my fruit before I eat dinner. For dinner, I usually tend to have a few different types of lightly-cooked vegetables like cauliflower and carrots, or collard greens and okra, along with a baked potato. I still eat meat, but not as often and not with any potatoes or other types of starches or complex carbohydrates.

Eating meat with rice, potatoes, bread, and any other kind of starch is what messes up our insides. This is because there are digestive protein acids and digestive complex carbohydrate alkalies in your stomach. When you eat meat, the digestive protein acids released in your stomach attack this protein to digest it. When you eat a starch or complex carbohydrate, the digestive complex carbohydrate alkalies in your stomach attack this food. If you eat meat (protein) and starch (a complex carbohydrate) together, the digestive acids and alkalies are both released and they actually nullify each other. Then the food you have eaten that is improperly combined sits in your stomach and takes much longer to digest — if at all! Even though I make sure to properly combine what I am eating, I have discovered that I can eat whatever I desire, as long as it is in moderation.

The point of all of this is, if you are still waiting for your healing, you need to realize you could be like me and not know everything. You need to get help from your doctors. Trust God to work through your doctors as you get all the help you can in this physical realm. You need all the faith you can use when you are going through an attack on your body, and you need all the help you can get from doctors, friends, and family. What you do not need to be doing is just waiting and consoling yourself with the hope of a miracle. And you certainly do not need to be wondering, "Well, I might not be operating in faith," when you consult and are following the advice of your physician. Never forget that if your faith was not strong enough to keep an attack on your body from coming against you in the first place, how are you going to believe for this attack to just disappear?

5

INTO RICH FULFILLMENT

When you are taking a stand of faith for your healing, be obedient and believe God to work through the chemotherapy, the radiation, or whatever treatments the doctors may recommend. Believe God to guide the minds and hands of the doctors working on your behalf. Believe God and take responsibility for doing whatever is physically possible to ensure your health. God will be with you through whatever you have to face. You cannot let the devil back you into a corner thinking, "Well, I am not going to make it." This is fear and 2 Timothy 1:7 says **...God has not given us a spirit of fear, but of power and of love and of a sound mind**. If you have any fear, it did not come from God. So, as my husband says, "You have no business with it."

Seek the guidance and revelation knowledge of the Holy Spirit. Ask that the eyes of your understanding be enlightened so you may make the right decisions. Pray the Holy Spirit reveals to you if there is anything you are doing or not doing to hinder the manifestation of your healing. Then honestly ask yourself, "Am I living my life as I should be unto the Lord?" Living right is a choice. There are all kinds of things you can be doing to hurt yourself. You could be killing yourself because you are walking in the flesh. Take some time for honest, *godly* introspection — *this is not the time to get caught up in guilt and condemnation.* Only Jesus was perfect — God does not expect you to be perfect. Jesus fulfilled the law of God so you do not have to be held in bondage by your past mistakes. Your job is to do your very best to maintain a holy lifestyle. If you realize you have made a mistake, then ask God for His forgiveness, receive His forgiveness by faith, and move on. If there are changes you need to make, then make them. Move on in whatever you need to be doing in acting responsibly toward your health.

You also need to make sure you are not harboring any unforgiveness. In Matthew 18:21-35, Mark 11:25-26, and Luke 6:37, the Bible very clearly commands us to forgive. Proverbs 3:1 says:

> **My son, do not forget my law,**
> **But let your heart keep my commands;**
> **For length of days and long life**
> **And peace they will add to you.**

God promises when you keep His commandments, **...length of days and long life and peace they will add to you**. If you are not a forgiving person, you are not keeping the law; you are forfeiting your promise of long life and peace. If you are not forgiving others and insist on harboring their offenses in your heart, all this unforgiveness, pain, and anger is bound to build up inside of you. This could be the reason why you may be experiencing an attack against your health. A lot of the time things happen to you because you are holding so much junk inside. If you do not get this junk out of you, then God cannot move on your behalf. You have a part to play. If you make up your mind that you are going to do what you are supposed to no matter what comes against you, you can know you are going to come out on top of any attack because you have the Word of God on your side. But you have got to first close every door as much as you know how, then go on and walk through this life. The enemy can attack you, but he cannot prevail if you are doing what you are supposed to do.

No matter how bad it looks, keep your focus on God's Word because it is power and it is life. You will find the Bible will sustain you when you are going through challenging times. Stir up the Word that is in you; talk to yourself, encourage yourself, and keep fighting. Just as King David encouraged himself in the Lord when his very life was threatened (1 Samuel 30:6), encourage yourself in the Lord. Psalm 103 records how David spoke to the Lord and himself in the midst of a trial, and this is exactly how I encouraged myself when it seemed there was nothing to be encouraged about:

> **Bless the LORD, O my soul;**
> **And all that is within me, bless His holy name!**
> **Bless the LORD, O my soul,**
> **And forget not all His benefits:**
> **Who forgives all your iniquities,**

Who heals all your diseases,
Who redeems your life from destruction,
Who crowns you with lovingkindness and
tender mercies,
Who satisfies your mouth with good things,
So that your youth is renewed like the eagle's.

I can personally assure you that God's Word works, but you have got to be strong and keep it stirred up inside of you. I had a very interesting experience which proves just how strong you have to remain — and that you cannot ever give up!

After my initial recovery from the cancerous tumor, I had to take an MRI every six months. When you go through a trauma like cancer, the doctors do not consider this condition as "healed," or in remission, until after five years have passed without any recurrence. Until that time, they rightfully insist on follow-up tests and check-ups. All the MRI's I had taken during the first four years following my initial recovery were just fine, and I was feeling progressively better and better. But then I went in for my regular MRI test and the doctors did not get back to me for a couple of weeks. When I finally did hear from them, they said there was something on my latest MRI which looked as if the lymphoma had come back. The doctor told me to get another MRI in three months. You can imagine how I felt and what I had to go through until it was time for my next MRI!

Yet I did not miss a beat. I taught "Successful Christian Living" every Tuesday afternoon and conducted a prayer meeting every Thursday evening at the church. But I had to talk to myself. I said, "God's Word is true. If I do not make it, it does not matter. I am going to go on teaching and conducting healing services even if I have to drag myself in there. Whatever I have to do to continue in God's Word and be obedient, I will do." I had to take this stand because the devil was telling me this was it. This kind of a doctor's report instantly makes you begin having pains all over your body. It is so real; you really feel as though this is it.

My mind was bombarded with negative thoughts, but praise God for His Word that I had programmed into my mind. I had to put 2 Corinthians 10:5 into practice and cast down the imaginations, arguments, reasoning, and every high thing that was trying to exalt itself above the knowledge of God. I had to cast all the negative thoughts out of my mind, replenishing and filling myself up with the Word of God. No matter what I heard, I would say, "Well, Jesus sent His Word and healed me. With Jesus' stripes, I am healed." I had to fight hard; I could not afford to get depressed. I had to keep coming to minister and pray for the sick even though the devil was telling me that I was not well. I told the devil, "I am still going to do it; it does not matter if I go up there and fall down, I am going to do whatever I have to do. I am presenting the Word of God, and the Word of God is true. So I will do it no matter what." This is the way you have to talk to yourself and the devil. You cannot think about what comes to your mind; you have to stay focused on the Word of God. I knew I could not let the devil take over my mind because he really would have turned this doctor's report into something drastic. Fear can bring sickness and disease upon your body, so you have to fight against fear.

People complain that faith does not make sense. Well, fear does not make any sense either! If you allow yourself to become afraid, what good does it do you? Satan will only have you running around scared. Fear will kill you a lot faster than any sickness or disease! Faith, however, is giving the Word of God precedence over anything that exalts itself above the knowledge of God. Despite how grim the doctor's report may be, God says by Jesus' stripes you were healed (1 Peter 2:24). Either you can believe God's Word and receive your healing by faith, or you can surrender to fear and death.

I thanked God every day for healing everything concerning my leg. It was a fight. I had to keep on saying, "I believe I am healed." I believed God and prayed:

> "Lord, You are in this with me. You would never leave me nor forsake me. There is no temptation taken me but such as is common to man, but You are faithful. You will not allow me to be tempted, tried, or tested above all that I am able, but will with that temptation, test, or trial, make a way of escape for me that I may be able to bear it."

I would read some of my favorite accounts of healings found in the Old Testament, because God has always been in the healing business. I would read in Numbers 12:1-16 about God's mercy toward Aaron and Miriam despite their dissension with Moses. In Numbers 21:4-9, I would read about the enduring mercy of God toward the Israelites. In 2 Kings 5:1-14, I was reminded of how God healed Naaman's leprosy. Both 2 Kings 20:1-11 and 2 Chronicles 32:24-26 encouraged me with their story of Hezekiah being healed. These biblical accounts of Jehovah-rapha ("The God Who Heals You") greatly boosted my faith.

Then I would read in Matthew 8:5-13 about Jesus healing the centurion's servant. In Matthew 8:1-4, I would be reminded of how Jesus cleansed the leper. I read that Peter's mother-in-law was healed by Jesus in Matthew 8:14-15, and was encouraged by Matthew 9:1-8's story of Jesus forgiving and healing the paralytic. My faith was charged when I read in Matthew 9:27-31 about Jesus healing the two blind men. I would use Matthew 9:35-38 to remind myself of my Father's compassion for His scattered sheep and could see this same compassion in Mark 3:1-5, when Jesus suffered persecution for healing a man's withered hand on the Sabbath. It was exciting to read in Mark 5:25-34 of how the woman with the issue of blood was instantly healed when she touched Jesus' garment. In Mark 10:46-52, I would read of Jesus stopping to heal blind Bartimaeus, who just called out to Him. Luke 6:17-19 says Jesus healed a great multitude; and in Luke 9:10-11 I would read of Jesus healing all those who needed healing — this was such a blessing to me because no one was left out. Luke 13:10-13 records Jesus healing the woman with a spirit of infirmity for over 18 years, so I was encouraged to keep standing in faith. Jesus still is in the healing business. For Hebrews 13:8 says:

> **Jesus Christ is the same yesterday, today, and forever.**

Throughout this time, I was feeling pain all over my body. My leg even began to swell. But I kept right on confessing the Word and meeting all of my obligations within my family and the ministry. It turned out the devil was just playing tricks on my mind. When the report came back from the next MRI, the doctors realized the spot they saw was actually the metal on my hip replacement!

In John 10:10, Jesus lets us know Satan is a thief. If he cannot rob you of your health and very life, he will try to steal your peace and joy. There are people who have been healed, yet they are scared the sickness or disease which attacked them before is going to come back upon them. What peace and joy is there in that? I refuse to be afraid of that! My trust is in the Lord. He said in Psalm 91:16 with long life He will satisfy me. So I believe as long as I have done all I am supposed to do, there is no way Satan can destroy me.

Never forget these encouraging words given to us in 3 John 2, that helped sustain me:

**Beloved, I pray that you may prosper in all
things and be in health, just as your soul prospers.**

The Word of God got me through this terrible
attack on my health. The Word of God is what
keeps me going day by day. Knowing I have God's
Word, I do not have to go down to the level of how
I feel, but I can rise up to what I believe. I believe
God's Word, so it does not matter what the enemy
tries to bring against me because the Word of God
guarantees my victory.

You had better learn the Word while you are
well, strong, and able because there may come a time
when you are under attack and cannot get to your
Bible. Say you are in the hospital, on machines, and
all kinds of disorienting medication, you certainly
will not be able to read the Bible for yourself. I know;
I have been there. It is absolutely amazing how you
can have no symptoms in your body and then, the
moment the doctor tells you there is something
wrong in your body, it is like all hell breaks loose.
There is no letting up on your mind. Nothing can
calm your mind like the Word of God when you
know it is true. You really need to be full of God's
Word so you can fight back.

The scriptures given in Appendix II are the ones
I specifically used when I was going through this
attack on my body. As you can see, the Father has
filled His Word with so much to help us. Many of
these scriptures I memorized as a child simply
because I loved the way they sounded; I did not have

the foggiest idea what they meant! For example, I just loved this scripture from Romans 8:37:

> **Yet in all these things we are more than conquerors through Him who loved us.**

But at that time I was conquered by everything. I was scared of everything. I confessed this verse because it sounded good and was beautiful, but I did not know I was supposed to be applying it to my life. And I certainly had never learned how to apply it to my life. I was saying, "I am more than a conqueror," yet I looked like a loser.

This is what a lot of people do. They do not realize that you have to take the Word and really apply it by faith to your life. Then the Word will manifest in your life. This is what is called letting the written Word or *logos* become a reality or *rhema* in your life. Only then will you know that you know the reality of the power and life encompassed in the Word of God.

Psalm 66:10-12 reads:

> **For You, O God, have tested us;**
> **You have refined us as silver is refined.**
> **You brought us into the net;**
> **You laid affliction on our backs.**
> **You have caused men to ride over our heads;**
> **We went through fire and through water;**
> **But You brought us out to rich fulfillment.**

Your faith will be proven, but it is not God proving you because He is omniscient — He already knows what you are going to do. Satan is the one who will prove you. In the original Hebrew, there is both the permissive and the causative sense of the verb form. For some reason, scholars have translated such verses as these in the causative sense, when you can tell from other scripture witnesses the permissive sense is really the appropriate verb form. God allows things to happen, but He does not put things on you.

My husband explains that to build anything in your life, you must have an opposing force. Just as barbells and dumb bells are used to build physical muscles, temptations, trials, and tests are the "spiritual weights" God allows in order that you can and will be spiritually strengthened. God permits temptations to come in order to develop and mature you, and He is so good that He does not allow you to be tempted, tried, or tested beyond what you can handle. This, again, is why you must not necessarily rebel against every hardship. Every step up helps you to take another step up. You need to trust that God will prove true to His Word and not allow you to be tempted, tried, or tested above that which you are able to bear (1 Corinthians 10:13). Know with every temptation, trial, or test, His Word says *He has already provided a way of escape.* So stand your ground against any and every temptation, trial, and test while you seek the way of escape which God has already provided for you.

Verse 11 of Psalm 66 goes on to say **You brought us into the net; You laid affliction on our backs.** Again you can see God *allowed* or permitted you to be brought into the net and affliction to come upon you. But God is not the cause — He is your way of escape! **You have caused men to ride over our heads** [*allowed* them to ride over our heads]; **We went through fire and through water;** *but You brought us out to rich fulfillment. You brought us out* — God provided the way of escape! This is where I can truly say I am today. I certainly went through the fire and through the water, but God was with me and He brought me out into rich fulfillment.

Appendix I

PHYSICIANS' REPORTS

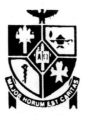

Saint John's Hospital and Health Center

Department of Radiation Oncology
Kenneth M. Tokita, M.D., Director
John Horns, M.D., Associate

March 7, 1991

William Taylor, M.D.
1760 Termino Ave., Suite 307
Long Beach, CA 90804

Re: BETTY PRICE #161606

Dear Bill,

Thank you very much for the elegance in coming down with Betty today.

She presents as an attractive, but unfortunate, 57 year old, black female with this history of lymphoma involving her lower abdomen. The history is certainly discouraging in that you had made this diagnosis back in May of last year, with a preceding one month history of discomfort. She apparently went on an airline trip and came back with marked swelling of her right leg. She apparently went promptly to you and subsequent very clear and careful examination revealed a mass in her right pelvis and subsequent biopsy was apparently consistent with lymphoma.

She was seen by medical oncology and, unfortunately, found it very difficult to buy into the program. Unfortunately, they read it as very negative and opted for a healing program, which is actually quite consistent with her husband's church. She actually has gotten along fairly well in the interim, but unfortunately recently her symptoms have increased. She has gotten increasing pain involving her entire right leg now, swelling in her right lower abdomen. She also has pain down the back of her leg and some mild swelling of that leg. She is increasingly anorexic.

Symptomatically, otherwise she has had no fever or chills, but she has had very definite sweats at night. She describes these as distinctly different from her menopausal hot flashes, as they are prolonged sweats and have been happening almost every night now.

MEDICATIONS: She is on 3 Percodan every 2-3 hours with Vistaril. She is also taking Halcion at night for sleep.

PAST MEDICAL HISTORY:

Allergies: None.

Illnesses: As above.

Medications: She is on Percodan, Vistaril and Motrin.

Surgery: She had the above mentioned biopsy in June of 1990. She also had a gluteal abscess in August of 1958 with no long term sequela.

Smoking: None.

Alcohol: None.

REVIEW OF SYSTEMS:
Remarkably clear, except for glasses, also the swelling that we described above, also some heartburn and also hemorrhoids in the past. Menstrually, she is Gravida V, para 4, AB 1, postmenopausal.

PHYSICAL EXAMINATION:
General: The patient presents as a middle aged, alert, attractive, black female who is very tired appearing, chronically ill appearing, sitting in a wheelchair and really unable to walk well because of the severe pain in her right leg. In general, she is a very sharp, very alert female who is very well aware of the seriousness of the situation.

Head: Normocephalic. Eyes: PERRLA. EOM and fields are intact. Fundi are within normal limits. There was no evidence of papilledema. Ears and nose: Unremarkable. Intraoral examination was dry, but otherwise unremarkable. Indirect nasopharyngoscopy and laryngoscopy are easily carried out and are unremarkable. There was no evidence of disease in Waldeyer's ring.

Neck: Supple without any palpable preauricular, digastric, cervical or supraclavicular adenopathy.

Axillae: Clear.

Chest: Remarkably clear on percussion and auscultation.

Spine: Straight and nontender to percussion.

Breasts: Symmetrical, easily examined without masses.

Heart: reveals sinus rhythm without murmur, taps or rubs.

Abdomen: Reveals a very definite, large mass in her right lower quadrant. It measures at least 15 x 15 cm, firm, feels fixed to the right pelvic sideway, extends up to the umbilicus and up to the midline. It does not appear to cross much over it. There is moderate tenderness on palpation, but I feel no other abdominal masses. Liver was down two fingerbreadths on maximal inspiration, percussed to a relatively normal 10 cm in the midclavicular line. The spleen was not palpable. No other masses were noted on palpation. The inguinal region reveals a fullness in the right groin, although I can't be sure exactly what that is. The left groin appears normal.

Pelvic: Examination was almost impossible with the pain she is having in her right leg.

Extremities: Reveal a moderate edema of the right leg, all the way down to her ankles. There was some mild edema on the left, but not as remarkable.

Neurologic: She was oriented X3. Cranial nerves II-XII are intact. Neuromuscular examination was weak throughout, but very weak in her right leg. Reflexes were symmetrical, 1+ in both legs with toes downgoing bilaterally. Sensory was grossly normal to touch, pain, proprioception and vibratory sense throughout.

IMPRESSION:
A 57 year old, black female with what I am sure is a very extensive lymphoma. She was a Stage II lymphoma back in June, but her more recent night sweats would make her at least a B and with what is being described, I would be very surprised if she wasn't a very advanced Stage II.

At any rate, the histology as read at Long Beach was a histiocytic lymphoma, which would make it very high grade.

RECOMMENDATIONS:
1. To see Pete as soon as possible – and thank you very much for seeing so promptly today in my office.

2. CT scan of her chest, upper abdomen and pelvis.

3. Blood tests as per you, Pete.

4. She really needs aggressive chemotherapy. There is no place for radiation right now, although if she does not respond as quickly as we might like, it may be meaningful to consider treating her pelvis and groin.

5. Steroids may be indicated right now because the pain is really getting excruciating and that may help relieve some of that.

At any rate, she understands how serious the situation is, but in a lymphoma, there is no way to know how she is going to do. She may do much better than we think, although there is obviously the very strong likelihood that she will not do well.

Thank you, Bill, for the elegance of escorting them down here and thank you, Pete, for seeing her in hopes that we can do something for her.

Sincerely,

Kenneth M. Tokita, M.D.
KT:cb

CC: Peter Boasberg, M.D.

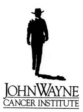

JOHN WAYNE
CANCER INSTITUTE

PETER D. BOASBERG, M.D., F.A.C.P.
Medical Oncology

2001 SANTA MONICA BLVD.
SUITE 1050
SANTA MONICA, CA 90404
310-998-3961
FAX 310-998-3965

January 2, 1997

Re: Betty R. Price

Dear Dr. Taylor:

When I first saw Mrs. Price, in the winter of 1991 and I found her very ill. She had
marked discomfort and weakness of her right leg and on exam, there was a large mass in
her lower abdomen. A CAT scan showed a 5 five inch pelvic mass that had grown into
the pelvic bones through the muscles and pushing the muscles, nerves and blood vessels of
the right leg. Biopsies showed evidence of spread of cancer to the marrow of the bones.
When she started chemotherapy, I was not optimistic that a cure was very likely. After
the first treatment, I was amazed at Mrs. Price's immediate and dramatic response with a
marked reduction in the tumor size and lessened pain and swelling allowing for greater
mobility. Within the two weeks, I could not feel the tumor at all! She continued through
the prescribed treatment and remained an excellent patient, always cooperative, cheerful
and fully involved. I was especially inspired with her quiet confidence that she would be
cured which I attributed to her strong faith in God. Now, much to my pleasure, I am
writing this narrative about this special woman who is no longer my patient for I believe
she is cured.

Respectfully,

Peter D. Boasberg, M.D., F.A.C.P.
Administrative Director, Medical Oncology
John Wayne Cancer Institute for Cancer Treatment and Research

AFFILIATED WITH SAINT JOHN'S HOSPITAL AND HEALTH CENTER SANTA MONICA, CA 90404

Appendix II

HEALING SCRIPTURES

HEALING SCRIPTURES

Exodus 15:26:

..."If you diligently heed the voice of the LORD your God and do what is right in His sight, give ear to His commandments and keep all His statutes, I will put [allow or permit] none of the diseases on you which I have brought [allowed or permitted] on the Egyptians. For I am the LORD who heals you."

Exodus 23:25:

"So you shall serve the LORD your God, and He will bless your bread and your water. And I will take sickness away from the midst of you."

Psalm 66:10-12:

For You, O God, have [allowed or permitted us to be] **tested us;**
You have [allowed or permitted us to be] **refined us as silver is refined.**
You [allowed or permitted us to be] **brought us into the net;**
You [allowed or permitted] **laid affliction on our backs.**
You have caused [allowed or permitted] **men to ride over our heads;**
We went through fire and through water;
But You brought us out to rich fulfillment.

Psalm 84:11:

> For the LORD God is a sun and shield;
> The LORD will give grace and glory;
> No good thing will He withhold
> From those who walk uprightly.

Psalm 91:7:

> A thousand may fall at your side,
> And ten thousand at your right hand;
> But it shall not come near you.

Psalm 91:10:

> No evil shall befall you,
> Nor shall any plague come near your dwelling.

Psalm 103:1-5:

> Bless the LORD, O my soul;
> And all that is within me, bless His holy name!
> Bless the LORD, O my soul,
> And forget not all His benefits:
> Who forgives all your iniquities,
> Who heals all your diseases,
> Who redeems your life from destruction,
> Who crowns you with lovingkindness and
>   tender mercies,
> Who satisfies your mouth with good things,
> So that your youth is renewed like the eagle's.

Psalm 107:20:

> He sent His word and healed them,
> And delivered them from their destructions.

Psalm 118:17:

> I shall not die, but live,
> And declare the works of the LORD.

Psalm 138:7-8:

> Though I walk in the midst of trouble, You will
>   revive me;
> You will stretch out Your hand
> Against the wrath of my enemies,
> And Your right hand will save me.
> The LORD will perfect that which concerns me;
> Your mercy, O LORD, endures forever;
> Do not forsake the works of Your hands.

Proverbs 3:1-5:

> My son, do not forget my law,
> But let your heart keep my commands;
> For length of days and long life
> And peace they will add to you.
> Let not mercy and truth forsake you;
> Bind them around your neck,
> Write them on the tablet of your heart,
> And so find favor and high esteem
> In the sight of God and man.

Trust in the LORD with all your heart,
And lean not on your own understanding.

Proverbs 3:24:

When you lie down, you will not be afraid;
Yes, you will lie down and your sleep will
be sweet.

Proverbs 4:4:

He also taught me, and said to me:
"Let your heart retain my words;
Keep my commands, and live."

Proverbs 4:20-23:

My son, give attention to my words;
Incline your ear to my sayings.
Do not let them depart from your eyes;
Keep them in the midst of your heart;
For they are life to those who find them,
And health to all their flesh.
Keep your heart with all diligence,
For out of it spring the issues of life.

Isaiah 53:4-5:

Surely He has borne our griefs
And carried our sorrows;
Yet we esteemed Him stricken,
Smitten by God, and afflicted.

But He was wounded for our transgressions,
He was bruised for our iniquities;
The chastisement for our peace was upon Him,
And by His stripes we are healed.

Jeremiah 30:17:

'For I will restore health to you
And heal you of your wounds,' says the LORD,
'Because they called you an outcast saying:
"This is Zion;
No one seeks her."'

Matthew 8:17:

That it might be fulfilled which was spoken
by Isaiah the prophet, saying:
"He Himself took our infirmities
And bore our sicknesses."

Mark 11:24:

"Therefore I say to you, whatever things you
ask when you pray, believe that you receive them,
and you will have them."

John 10:10:

"The thief does not come except to steal, and to
kill, and to destroy. I have come that they may have
life, and that they may have it more abundantly."

John 11:4:

When Jesus heard that, He said, "This sickness is not unto death, but for the glory of God, that the Son of God may be glorified through it."

Romans 8:11:

But if the Spirit of Him who raised Jesus from the dead dwells in you, He who raised Christ from the dead will also give life to your mortal bodies through His Spirit who dwells in you.

1 Corinthians 10:13:

No temptation has overtaken you except such as is common to man; but God is faithful, who will not allow you to be tempted beyond what you are able, but with the temptation will also make the way of escape, that you may be able to bear it.

2 Corinthians 4:18:

While we do not look at the things which are seen, but at the things which are not seen. For the things which are seen are temporary, but the things which are not seen are eternal.

2 Corinthians 10:4-5:

For the weapons of our warfare are not carnal but mighty in God for pulling down strongholds,
casting down arguments and every high thing that exalts itself against the knowledge of God, bringing every thought into captivity to the obedience of Christ.

Philippians 4:13:

I can do all things through Christ who strengthens me.

Hebrews 13:5:

Let your conduct be without covetousness; be content with such things as you have. For He Himself has said, "I will never leave you nor forsake you."

Hebrews 13:8:

Jesus Christ is the same yesterday, today, and forever.

James 1:1-3:

James, a bondservant of God and of the Lord Jesus Christ,
To the twelve tribes which are scattered abroad: Greetings.

My brethren, count it all joy when you fall into various trials,

knowing that the testing [proving] of your faith produces patience.

James 5:14-15:

Is anyone among you sick? Let him call for the elders of the church, and let them pray over him, anointing him with oil in the name of the Lord.

And the prayer of faith will save the sick, and the Lord will raise him up. And if he has committed sins, he will be forgiven.

1 Peter 2:24:

Who Himself bore our sins in His own body on the tree, that we, having died to sins, might live for righteousness — by whose stripes you were healed.

1 John 3:21-22:

Beloved, if our heart does not condemn us, we have confidence toward God.

And whatever we ask we receive from Him, because we keep His commandments and do those things that are pleasing in His sight.

Appendix II

1 John 5:4:

For whatever is born of God overcomes the world. And this is the victory that has overcome the world — our faith.

1 John 5:14-15:

Now this is the confidence that we have in Him, that if we ask anything according to His will, He hears us.

And if we know that He hears us, whatever we ask, we know that we have the petitions that we have asked of Him.

3 John 2:

Beloved, I pray that you may prosper in all things and be in health, just as your soul prospers.

Jude 1:20:

But you, beloved, building yourselves up on your most holy faith, praying in the Holy Spirit.

Revelation 12:11:

"And they overcame him by the blood of the Lamb and by the word of their testimony, and they did not love their lives to the death."

79

Appendix III

PRAYERS

by

Dr. Betty R. Price

PRAYERS
by Dr. Betty R. Price

Prayer involves a personal relationship with God which you enter into when you receive Jesus Christ as your personal Savior and Lord. If you have not accepted Jesus Christ as your personal Savior and Lord, then you need to. John 14:6 tells us Jesus is the way, the truth, and the life. No one comes to the Father except through Jesus. If you would like to establish a one-on-one relationship with the Father through Jesus Christ, His only begotten Son, then I encourage you to pray the following prayer of salvation:

Dear God:

Your Word says, in Romans 10:9-10, if I confess Your Son, Jesus, as my Savior and Lord, and believe in my heart that You raised Him from the dead, I will be saved. "For with the heart one believes unto righteousness and with the mouth confession is made unto salvation."

I believe Jesus Christ is Your Son, and that He was sent into the world as Savior to redeem my life. I believe He died for me, and that He was raised from the dead for my justification. Jesus, be the Lord over my life. I confess You now as my Savior and Lord. I believe with my heart that according to the Word, I have now become the righteousness of God in Christ, and I am now saved.

Thank You, Father, in Jesus' name. Amen.

If you are not sure how to pray, or need help getting started, I suggest you start with the Word of God. Since God honors His Word, you can be confident your prayers are heard by the Father and are effective when you pray God's Word (1 John 5:14-15). From there, begin to express your own, unique self. Spend time talking to your Father. He loves you, and the time you spend in prayer is a reflection of your love for Him.

A PRAYER FOR HEALING

Father God,

I thank You that Jesus Himself took my infirmities and bore my sicknesses, by whose stripes I am healed. For Jesus bore my sins in His own body on a tree that I, being dead to sins, might live for righteousness. Jesus redeemed me from the curse of the law having become a curse for me; for it is written, "Cursed is everyone who hangs on a tree."

Thank You, Father, that the same spirit who raised Jesus from the dead dwells in me, and I am being made alive in my mortal body by this same Spirit. Thank You that I have overcome sickness and disease by the blood of the Lamb and the word of my testimony.

Thank You that the joy of the Lord is my strength, and that the joy of the Lord remains in me. So I rejoice in the Lord always.

I give You praise and thanksgiving that neither death nor life, nor angels nor principalities nor powers, nor things present nor things to come, nor height nor depth, nor any other created thing shall be able to separate me from the love of God which is in Christ Jesus. In Him, Jesus Christ, I live, move, and have my being.

I thank You that all things work together for my good. For the eyes of the Lord are on the righteous, and His ears are open to their prayers. I praise You, Father, for delivering me from the power of darkness and conveying me into the kingdom of Jesus Christ. Satan no longer holds any dominion over me. I am more than a conqueror through Him who loves me; and since God is for me, who can be successfully against me?

Thank You, Father, that I am not anxious about anything. In everything, by prayer and supplication with thanksgiving, I have let my requests be made known to You. Therefore, I have Your peace, which surpasses all understanding and guards my heart and mind through Jesus Christ. So I hold fast the confession of my hope without wavering because I know God is faithful to keep His promises. My God supplies all my needs according to His riches in glory by Christ Jesus.

And Father, this is the confidence that I have in You. The Word declares that if I ask anything according to Your will, You hear me. And I know that if You hear me, I have the petitions I ask of You.

So I give You all the praise, glory, and honor in advance for all You have done to bring complete healing and restoration to my body and every aspect of my life and family.

In Jesus' name. Amen.

PRAYER FOR YOUR DOCTORS

Dear Father God,

*I give You praise, glory, and thanksgiving for Your great love for me. I thank You that You are an ever-present help in time of need. I thank You that You are the Healer and that You know all concerning this condition trying to threaten the wholeness of my body and the soundness of mind You gave me when I accepted Jesus as my personal Lord and Savior. I thank You that by Jesus' stripes I **am** healed. I pray that You, as my Chief Physician, will direct my doctors (state their names) in my (operation, treatments, tests, therapy). Give them the wisdom to perform my (operation, treatments, tests, therapy) successfully. Assist them in helping me to completely recover from this attack on my body. Reveal to my doctors all the means by which they can aid in the complete healing and restoration of my body.*

May my doctors have clarity of mind as they examine, perform, and review my (treatments, tests, therapy). May they have the insight, personal strength, sensitivity, patience, and endurance needed to help see me through this time. I bind the spirits of confusion, deception, fear, and infirmity in the Name of Jesus.

I thank You in advance for a speedy and painless recovery. Thank You for peace of mind and comfort in my body. Thank You for Your help in enabling me to remain a true witness for Jesus Christ. I thank You for the victory now, in advance, for there is nothing too hard or too big for You. May my doctors come to have a greater

revelation of the reality of Jesus Christ as you turn what
the devil meant for my harm into victory for the praise and
glory of Your name.

I covenant with You that You alone will receive all the
praise and glory for my healing and complete restoration.

I pray this prayer in the mighty name of Jesus, my
Lord and Savior. Amen.

Appendix IV

THE PERSONALITY
OF CANCER

by

William F. Taylor, M.D.

THE PERSONALITY OF CANCER
by William F. Taylor, M.D.

Satan, the god of this world, states in the 14th chapter of Isaiah:

> ...I will ascend to heaven; I will exalt my throne above the stars of God; I will sit upon the mount of assembly in the uttermost north.
> I will ascend above the heights of the clouds; I will make myself like the Most High.
>
> Isaiah 14:13-14
> (The Amplified Bible)

Such is the pronouncement made by cancer as it seeks to displace, disfigure, and utterly destroy its host. Most organisms that partake of a host develop symbiotic relationships where both the host and the parasitic invaders are able to enjoy their relationship without the destruction of either. But the entity we call cancer exudes a type of occupancy that takes authority and dominion over the host it has invaded. The aim of a cancer is to steal, kill, and destroy. Doesn't this bear a striking resemblance to the intent of Satan? You bet it does! (John 10:10). Satan is, in fact, the entity behind the disease called cancer — just as he is the culprit behind all sickness, disease, and most human ills.

The term "cancer" refers to a diverse collection of over 100 forms of this malady, that all have in common a loss of the normal orderly mechanisms that regulate cell growth. A mutation in nearly any cell in the body can result in cellular chaos, ultimately manifesting itself as a malignant tumor that grows in an uncontrolled fashion, invading and destroying surrounding normal tissue.

The human body is comprised of over 30 trillion cells. Each one of these cells remains distinct, yet each cell is dependent and interdependent upon the others. As cells become specialized, they form organs. These organs sub-specialize and produce specific substances which benefit the entire body. The body's organs also link together to form what we call "systems." For example, the cardiovascular system is comprised of the heart and its associative arteries, veins, and capillaries. Just as each cell and each organ remains distinct yet interconnected, each bodily system is distinct yet interdependent on all of the other bodily systems in order for the entire body to function properly. This is the rhythm of life and it typifies the wonderful, God-given creation called the human being.

Psalm 139:14 states we are awesomely and wonderfully made. This splendor does not end with only the anatomy of the body. Into this marvelous structure, the Lord has placed an intricate and powerful ally — the awesome human immune system. The immune system is the body's principal defense mechanism against disease. This elaborate system is vibrant, containing a network or plethora of specialized "killer" cells. These cellular members may remain small in number, particularly if the body is not threatened. But when war is waged against the body, these cells can increase from 10,000 to over 100,000 killer cells. Each "killer" cell is ready and able to wage war. If this war continues, the body is able to shift into another gear by converting ordinary cells into *"killing machines."* In other words, the immune system tailors its offense to the type of intruder by releasing different amounts and types of white blood cells.

Thus the body sustains life by expressing a pattern of living that is consistent with godly principles. Each cell has its own specialized function, while joining with other cells to accomplish an ultimate purpose. Beauty lies in the ability of each cell to maintain its own distinct identity while working with other cells to accomplish a goal that is beneficial to the entire body as a whole. Complete harmony, peace, and unity within and amongst each and every cell produces a healthy body.

Interestingly enough, this same principle of the individual joining, cooperating, and working together with others for the greater good of all is how God envisions all the individual members of the Body of Christ to work together as one healthy, viable body. In 1 Corinthians 12:12-27, the Spirit of God, through the writings of the apostle Paul, elaborates on this principle:

> For as the body is one and has many members, but all the members of that one body, being many, are one body, so also is Christ.
>
> For by one Spirit we were all baptized into one body — whether Jews or Greeks, whether slaves or free — and have all been made to drink into one Spirit.
>
> For in fact the body is not one member but many.
>
> If the foot should say, "Because I am not a hand, I am not of the body," is it therefore not of the body?
>
> And if the ear should say, "Because I am not an eye, I am not of the body," is it therefore not of the body?
>
> If the whole body were an eye, where would be the hearing? If the whole were hearing, where would be the smelling?
>
> But now God has set the members, each one of them, in the body just as He pleased.
>
> And if they were all one member, where would the body be?
>
> But now indeed there are many members, yet one body.
>
> And the eye cannot say to the hand, "I have no need of you"; nor again the head to the feet, "I have no need of you."
>
> No, much rather, those members of the body which seem to be weaker are necessary.
>
> And those members of the body which we think to be less honorable, on these we bestow greater honor; and our unpresentable parts have greater modesty,

> but our presentable parts have no need. But
> God composed the body, having given greater
> honor to that part which lacks it,
> that there should be no schism in the body,
> but that the members should have the same care
> for one another.
> And if one member suffers, all the members
> suffer with it; or if one member is honored, all the
> members rejoice with it.
> Now you are the body of Christ, and members
> individually.

As long as each individual cell in the human
body maintains its own distinct identity while working
with other cells for the greater good of the entire body,
we will see our Savior's spiritual plan of salvation
resulting in wholeness, completeness, wellness,
unity, and peace expressed through the physical
manifestation of divine health.

A cancer begins when a cell breaks free from the
normal bodily mechanisms controlling its growth
and spread. Satan's declaration in Isaiah 14:13-14, **I
will make myself like the Most High,** typifies the
defiance an abhorrent cell personifies. This scenario
is played out initially in a few cells and ultimately
spreads to many. **A little leaven leavens the whole
lump** (Galatians 5:9). As a result, the orderly, obedient
cellular activity previously present in the normal
person's body suddenly changes.

A small mutinous group of cells, having thrown
off the body's system of control or restraint that
causes them to function normally, begin "to do their
own thing." They are no longer interested in playing

by the rules or operating in the spirit of unity. These cells become rogues, thieves, renegades, outlaws. They are selfish, often suicidal, and bent on destruction. Their physical appearance even changes as they take on the intent of their master, Satan.

Under the microscope, cancer cells look bizarre and act accordingly. The restraint to control their growth has been lost, so they multiply and divide without regard or concern for the rest of the body. These outlaw cells divide so rapidly and voluminously they outstrip their blood supply and commit hara-kiri (a Japanese form of ritualistic suicide). As I have indicated before, the aim of these cancerous cells is to steal, kill and destroy — even at their own expense. So they violate all the normal bodily relationships, wreaking havoc as they go.

What causes a normal, God-fearing cell to become a monstrous cancer cell? It is known by science and medicine that the delicate heart or nucleus of the normal cell, where the genes and chromosomes are located, changes. A mutation occurs, resulting in a change in the genetic make-up of the cell. Once this mutation has occurred, life is never the same. If something is not done to alter or halt the mutation, this assault goes on unchecked until there is a symptom that is painful or sizable enough to get the attention of the host (or person).

According to an article published in the December 23, 1996 issue of *Newsweek* magazine, entitled "The Cancer Killer" by Sharon Begley, science has discovered that gene p53 is "... a cell's most elegant defender....

It stops tumors before they grow. But if damaged, it is involved in 60 percent of cancers." In other words, according to this informative article, the p53 gene not only helps to keep tumors from forming, but it also helps to prevent a damaged cell from growing into a malignant tumor. However, if this gene itself is damaged in some way, it ceases to be a defender of the cell and can actually become a disease producer causing cancers. Think what science can do toward cancer prevention with this knowledge.

Currently, there are several signs which are generally accepted as *possible* warning signs of cancer. It is important to note that the occurrence of any of these signs does not necessarily have to be an indication of cancer; however, the presence of any one of these symptoms should receive immediate medical attention:

1). Unexplained weight loss
2). Unusual bleeding
3). A sore which does not heal
4). Unexplained pain
5). Night sweats
6). Weakness
7). Unexplained lumps, sometimes a mass with an unusual color change
8). A change in bowel habits

Many times, the Holy Spirit will prompt the person to seek help. Often for the Word-knowledge Christian, denial will set in with an attempt to either underplay the set of symptoms or spiritualize them by saying, "I am standing for my healing." In reality, most often what has happened is that fear has gripped the person into not seeking help or even discussing it (men are often more guilty of this than women).

But the dye has been cast. Sometimes weeks, months, or even years may pass before the symptoms worsen. In extreme cases, either a loss of a bodily function occurs or the cancerous mass may break open the skin exuding a foul discharge. The enemy may compound the assault by enabling the cells to break free from the tumor mass and begin traveling to distal sites in the body. This process is called metastasis. The tumor load itself, sometimes being phenomenal, can also cause havoc by its sheer size. If treatment (such as chemotherapy, radiation, or surgery) is not initiated, the bulky tumor can cause an overload, a disruption in function, or the release of toxins leading to multi-system failure and ultimately death.

But I have good news! Deuteronomy 28 says if we obey the voice of the Lord (that is, be sensitive to the leading of the Holy Spirit) and do as He commands us (in other words, "Be a doer of the Word," as admonished in James 1:22), then the Lord will cause His blessings of health and prosperity to come upon us. So, yes, cancer and like diseases exist, but they do not have to exist in you! Why? Because the doer of the Word is blessed! But blessings can be conditional, which is why you have to examine yourself to be sure you are doing all God has commanded you to do in His Word. For example, 1 Corinthians 11:29-30 says:

> For he who eats and drinks in an unworthy manner eats and drinks judgment to himself, not discerning the Lord's body.
> For this reason many are weak and sick among you, and many sleep.

For this reason, many are weak and sick among you, and many sleep. For what reason? **For not discerning the Lord's body.** But how many Christians truly recognize they are the Lord's body and how they are to properly care for the physical body they have been given? This is why God says in Hosea 4:6 **"My people are destroyed for lack of knowledge."** Part of doing all God has commanded you to do is knowing and adhering to what it takes to properly care for the awesome gift you have been given in the form of a physical, human body. The following factors have led too many Christians, despite having a knowledge of the Word of God, to fall prey to the likes of cancer:

a). Poor nutrition

b). Poor water intake

c). Poor bowel care

d). Maintaining a worldly lifestyle

e). Mind not renewed with the Word of God

f). Stress and unforgiveness

g). Flagrant disobedience of either natural or spiritual laws (or both!)

Though scientists project thousands of cancer patients in the United States will die annually, there have been striking reductions in death from some cancers, specifically Hodgkin's disease, Burkitt's lymphoma, testicular cancer, cancer of certain bones and muscles, and many that affect children. *Prevention is the key.* Research reveals that thirty percent of all cancers may be caused by smoking, with nearly an equal percentage spurred on either by one's lifestyle, dietary practices, or lack of exercise.

Part of a successful cancer prevention program includes thorough medical testing. Knowledge of what medical tests you should request from your doctor is key to ensuring that you have all the information necessary to make the right decisions concerning your health. Since managed health care emphasizes cost containment, you must know what to ask for when you see your physician. Both males and females should insist on having the following tests:

1). A chemistry panel called "Chem 20" — a battery of 20 blood tests

2). A complete blood count with differential

3). A urinalysis

4). An EKG or electrocardiogram or heart tracing

5). A thyroid profile

6). An RPR to R/O syphilis or herpes, hepatitis, profile and HIV, if you are sexually active, and

7). A baseline chest x-ray.

Each woman should have a pap smear and a mammogram within the time sequence determined by her specific medical history. Each male, especially 40 and above, should have a digital rectal exam and a blood test called a Prostate Specific Antigen (PSA). A yearly eye exam to evaluate visual acuity and measurement of eye pressure to rule out glaucoma is important. Periodic dental examinations also aide in determining your overall health.

Lastly, the Word of God declares that the power of life and death is in the tongue (Proverbs 18:21). So make daily confessions over your life that are consistent with the Word of God. For example:

"I am free from the curse of the law (Galatians 3:13) and by His stripes I am healed (1 Peter 2:24).
"I am covered by the blood of Jesus (Colossians 1:14) and no weapon formed against me shall prosper" (Isaiah 54:17).

Realizing since the power of life and death lies in the tongue, and the tongue is essential for swallowing, it naturally follows that proper nutrition also plays a powerful part in your health. Remember, be a doer of the Word by watching what you swallow!

Keep in mind also that Romans 12:1 says your body is to be a *living* sacrifice — the Father deems it only reasonable that you properly care for your body, as well as your spirit, and your soul. El Shaddai, the God who is More Than Enough, has said in Psalm 91:14-16:

> "Because he has set his love upon Me,
>   therefore will I deliver him;
> I will set him on high, because he has known
>   My name.
> He shall call upon Me, and I will answer him;
> I will be with him in trouble;
> I will deliver him and honor him.
> With long life I will satisfy him,
> And show him My salvation."

DR. WILLIAM F. TAYLOR *has been practicing Internal Medicine since 1979. He received his Bachelor of Arts degree from Dillard University, a Master of Science Degree from Texas Southern University, and his medical degree from the School of Medicine at Temple University in Philadelphia, PA. His internship and residency were done at the University of Southern California Medical Center in*

Los Angeles, and he has broadened his experience with specialty work at Osler Medical Service, Johns Hopkins Hospital, Harvard University, and the Cleveland Clinic.

Dr. Taylor is on the staffs and associated with Long Beach Community Hospital, Robert F. Kennedy Medical Center, and Bellflower General Hospital — all located in Los Angeles County.

He is a graduate of the Crenshaw Christian Center Ministry Training Institute and serves as President of the CCCMTI Alumni Association. Called to the ministry offices of Evangelist and Teacher, Dr. Taylor — a popular speaker — ministers the Word of God by embodying biblical knowledge coupled with medical acumen. His approach to medicine is enhanced by his spiritual philosophy, and he views the physical, emotional, and spiritual well-being of the human state as being intricately tied together.

Recognizing that man at his core is ultimately a spiritual being existing in a physical body, and that physical ills have a spiritual origin, Dr. Taylor has equipped himself with the knowledge of the Word of God to better serve the medical needs of his patients. His personal philosophy embodies the essence of the Holy Spirit which declares that the hand of God touching the hand of man becomes the "Prescription for Healing."

Appendix V

PICTURES

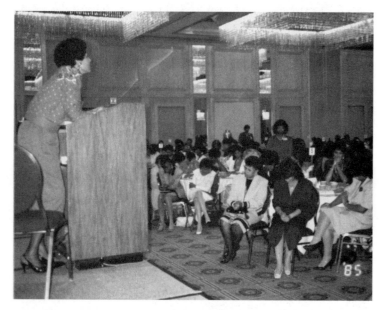

October 1990, "Wisdom From Above" luncheon where Dr. Betty informed the ladies of the attack of cancer.

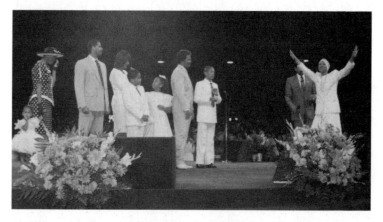

Resurrection Day 1991, in the FaithDome. Dr. Betty returns to church after a long absence.

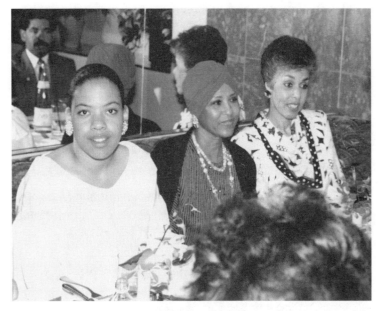

Secretaries' Day, April, 1991. Despite not being able to eat and a swollen face, Dr. Betty enjoyed a laugh with the church secretaries.

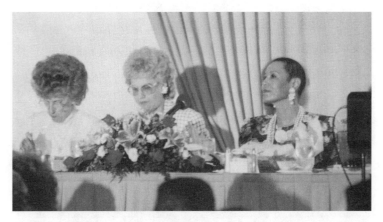

End of 1991, Dr. Betty as guest speaker at a women's luncheon.

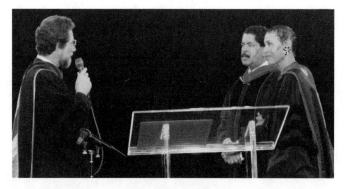

1991, in the FaithDome. Dr. Betty receiving her Honorary Doctor of Divinity degree from Friends International University.

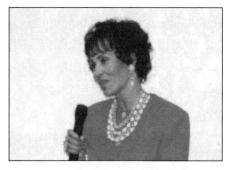

1993, Dr. Betty well on the mend, addressing Crenshaw Christian Center's Seniors' Fellowship.

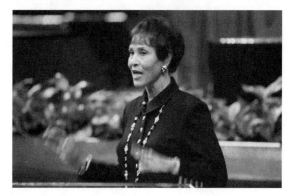

1996 CCC Women's Convention, keynote speaker Dr. Betty addressing the audience.

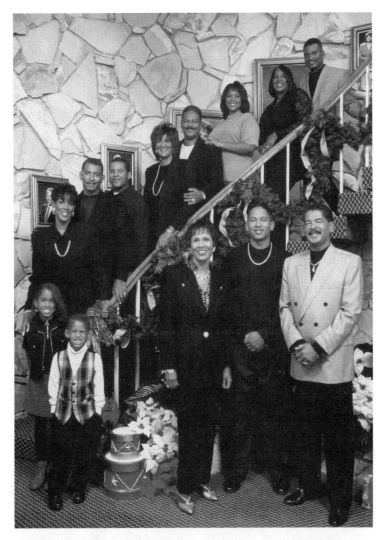

Christmas 1996, the Price Family (pictured R-L): Dr. Frederick K.C. Price; Frederick K. Price; Dr. Betty R. Price; Allen L. Crabbe, III; Nicole D. Crabbe; Cheryl A. Crabbe and Allen L. Crabbe, Jr.; Alan M. Evans; Angela M. Evans and A. Michael Evans, Jr.; Adrian M. Evans; Stephanie Buchanan and Danon Buchanan.

BOOKS BY FREDERICK K.C. PRICE, PH.D.
(continued)

THE VICTORIOUS, OVERCOMING LIFE
(A Verse-by-Verse Study of the Book of Colossians)

A NEW LAW FOR A NEW PEOPLE

THE FAITHFULNESS OF GOD

THE PROMISED LAND
(A New Era for the Body of Christ)

THREE KEYS TO POSITIVE CONFESSION

THE WAY, THE WALK,
AND THE WARFARE OF THE BELIEVER
(A Verse-by-Verse Study of the Book of Ephesians)

BEWARE! THE LIES OF SATAN

TESTING THE SPIRITS

THE CHASTENING OF THE LORD

IDENTIFIED WITH CHRIST:
A Complete Cycle From Defeat to Victory

THE CHRISTIAN FAMILY:
Practical Insight for Family Living
(formerly MARRIAGE AND THE FAMILY)

THE HOLY SPIRIT:
THE HELPER WE ALL NEED

FIVE LITTLE FOXES OF FAITH

Available from your local bookstore

For a complete list of books and tapes by
Dr. Frederick K.C. Price, and Dr. Betty R. Price, write:

Drs. Fred and Betty Price
Crenshaw Christian Center
P.O. Box 90000
Los Angeles CA 90009

BOOKS BY BETTY R. PRICE, D.D.

THROUGH THE FIRE AND THROUGH THE WATER
My Triumph Over Cancer

STANDING BY GOD'S MAN

BOOKS BY FREDERICK K.C. PRICE, PH.D.

HIGH FINANCE
God's Financial Plan: Tithes and Offerings

HOW FAITH WORKS
(In English and Spanish)

IS HEALING FOR ALL?

HOW TO OBTAIN STRONG FAITH
Six Principles

NOW FAITH IS

THE HOLY SPIRIT —
The Missing Ingredient

FAITH, FOOLISHNESS, OR PRESUMPTION?

THANK GOD FOR EVERYTHING?

HOW TO BELIEVE GOD FOR A MATE

LIVING IN THE REALM OF THE SPIRIT

THE ORIGIN OF SATAN

CONCERNING THEM WHICH ARE ASLEEP

HOMOSEXUALITY
State of Birth or State of Mind?

PROSPERITY ON GOD'S TERMS

WALKING IN GOD'S WORD
Through His Promises

PRACTICAL SUGGESTIONS FOR SUCCESSFUL MINISTRY

NAME IT AND CLAIM IT!
The Power of Positive Confession

(continued on next page)